THE LITTLE FOOD BOOK

you are what you eat

To: Jon

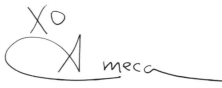

BY CRAIG SAMS

who always wants to know about what is in everything he eats.

XO
A meca

disinformation

The author and publishers have made every effort to ensure
the accuracy of the information in the book at the time of
going to press. However, they cannot accept any responsibility
for any loss, injury or inconvenience resulting from the use of
information contained in this guide.

disinformation

CREDITS

To Margaret Sams, whose
commitment to wholesome
food gave me such a good
start in life

Editor: Alastair Sawday

Project editors: Anne Sullivan, Sorrel Everton,
Jacob Rosette and Patrick Neighly

Design: Anne Marie Horne

Original illustrations: David Atkinson

Other illustrations: © 1995 Zedcor, Inc.

Project assistants: Jason Louv, Maya Shmuter
and Ralph Bernardo

Printed in USA

4

CONTENTS

INTRODUCTION

It was hepatitis, ironically, that gave me my first awareness of the importance of food to health. In 1965, travelling from India to Afghanistan, I developed hepatitis and was left at a low ebb. After following a macrobiotic diet, I recovered completely. In February 1966 I made a trip to New York to visit the macrobiotic bookshop on 5th Avenue. When I took some books to the cash register a rather morose woman told me that I couldn't buy them. They were awaiting a decision from the FBI before they could sell books again! At the instigation of the American Medical Association, the FBI had entered the shop and taken away books to see if they broke the law. They did. The books suggested that cancer could be prevented – even cured – by healthy eating. These were sufficiently serious offenses to justify the removal of the books. They were subsequently burned. The bookshop closed soon after and many shocked members of the small New York macrobiotic community moved to Chico, a town in northern California.

Such vehement reactions to macrobiotics were an extended attack that implied quasi-terrorist attributes to people who believed that "you are what you eat." It was a depressing moment, especially for anyone who had experienced the happiness that comes from vigorous good health based on a balanced diet of wholesome natural foods. Against the background of the Vietnam War, eating a macrobiotic diet became a political statement – one that was adopted by large numbers of my generation. The same evening as my visit to the bookshop, I also visited the Paradox, a macrobiotic restaurant in the East Village, and it was then I decided to change the plans for my life. I decided to open a macrobiotic restaurant in London, which I did in 1967.

As with so many ideas of the 1960s, macrobiotics, natural foods, healthy eating and organic living are no longer considered "lunatic fringe." Today the Harvard School of Public Health even suggests macrobiotics to avoid increasing obesity and diet-related disease. That little group of macrobiotics who moved to Chico set up a food company called Chico-San to distribute brown rice and similar foods. In 1998 Heinz bought it to give them entry into the organic food market in the USA. The expenditure on complementary and alternative healthcare in the US now exceeds spending on surgery and pharmaceuticals. Many doctors now have qualifications in nutrition, homeopathy and other therapies. They need them to be able to offer their patients a more holistic and preventative approach to health.

Since adopting a macrobiotic diet I have not needed a doctor and have taken no prescription drug. I have been ill at times but have learned to respect the importance of a healthy digestive system. My children have grown up with stronger constitutions and straighter teeth than I have. To me they are living proof that a diet that includes occasional meat and dairy products, and is weighted strongly towards whole grains and vegetables, can support health and strength. My grandchildren's physical robustness and balanced dispositions indicate that, notwithstanding Darwin, acquired characteristics can be inherited. We have the power to evolve in whatever direction we choose and what we eat can exercise a profound influence on us at the chromosomal level. We know that bad nutrition can lead to physical degeneration and that this can be inherited – the children of diabetics are more likely to develop diabetes. It follows that the children of healthy parents will be less likely to develop chronic illness.

The political attacks on macrobiotics taught me to regard the opinions of experts and government officials with a healthy scepticism. Over the years I've read that researchers and scientists have proved that white bread is better for you than wholegrain, that cancer is caused by a virus, that once we map the human genome we can cure all diseases, that without sugar we will lack energy and that meat is the best protein. Food, and its influence on physical and mental well-being, has been at the center of my business career and my personal life. Sometimes I may have been a bit fanatical. But "fanum" means "temple" and my body is my temple. I have looked extensively within and come to understand, through intuition, experience and study of the observations of others, how it works and how to keep it working well. I find it hard to accept science when it runs counter to my intuition and experience. But science, too, is beginning to take a more holistic view.

The world's diet is getting worse and better simultaneously. Every day, another four McDonald's restaurants open somewhere in the world – harbingers of a diet and lifestyle that leads inexorably to obesity. The diseases that arise from obesity and digestive malfunction are increasing as a modern, fast food diet displaces traditional ways of eating around the world. Yet, the numbers who go to bed hungry are still near one sixth of the world's population.

Nonetheless, every day more people choose to step off the junk food treadmill and enjoy a form of personal freedom. When they do so, the infrastructure that provides organic, natural and wholesome food expands a little bit more. Despite government policy that still bends to powerful pharmaceutical, medical and chemical interests, a new consensus about how and what we should eat, what is and isn't safe, is emerging. It is growing in the ever-crucial marketplace, and I am filled with optimism.

This little book will, I hope, contribute to that emerging consensus. It tackles key issues like nutrition, the politics of food and the mainsprings of health. If we all ate with an awareness of the importance of our food choices, there would be more health and justice on this crowded planet. With justice comes peace – the ultimate goal of civilization.

Craig Sams - author

HOW TO USE THIS BOOK

Dip in and out if you wish; take a subject at a time. Each chapter is short and to the point – however vast the subject – and aims to provoke you, both emotionally and intellectually. Do read further; the book symbol at the end of some chapters refers you to books and websites that go more deeply into the subjects, though the views expressed here don't necessarily represent the views of those books.

Better still, try reading it all at one or two sittings; the ideas, held together in your memory, will form a powerful whole. For that is the core message of this book: we cannot consider "food" in isolation. It is linked to far greater global issues. The book is divided loosely into five sections: general issues; food and big business; food and farming; food and nutrition, and thoughts to ponder. The range of issues is broad but they are all far too important not to be considered, as we hope you will see.

"When the sun rises, I go to work
When the sun goes down, I take my rest
I dig the well from which I drink
I farm the soil that yields my food,
I share creation, Kings can do no more."

Anonymous (Chinese, 2500BC)

POP TARTS, DING DONGS, TWINKIES AND CIVILIZATION

our world today

The rise in the total level of wealth and education in the world has been dramatic throughout the 20th century – despite two world wars. More people have more money and more valuable property than ever before. Secondary education is almost universal, university education widespread. Growing inequalities may mar the picture, but the level of wealth enjoyed by the large numbers of "haves" greatly exceeds anything in the past. Even many "have-nots" may still have proper sanitation and televisions and can choose to afford highly taxed products like alcohol and cigarettes.

This overall wealth has brought huge benefits. The air we breathe is much cleaner than it was when coal was routinely burned by industry and in the home and when lead in fuel was standard. The food we eat is free of many of the worst additives and adulterants that were once permitted. The water we drink conforms to new, more rigorous standards. Rivers are cleaner. Emphasis on safety in the workplace, in cars and in airplanes makes work and travel less likely to cause death or disability. The value society places on human life encourages us, as our individual and collective net worth increases, to improve our living conditions and invest to minimize the risk of threats to life.

So what on earth has gone wrong with our food? Food-related deaths exceed by many

What on earth has gone wrong with our food?

times deaths from car accidents and the rate is escalating. Diabetes, heart disease, obesity and cancer all point to a depressingly awful quality of life for increasing numbers of young people as they carry these (often) food-related diseases into adulthood. When we look at the range of what we eat, there has been an explosion of variety and sophistication, with "world fusion" cuisine as an expected norm. Yet there has been a parallel surge in nutritionally poor, unsafe food.

Candy was once a luxury and occasional treat. Now chocolate bars, doughnuts and Twinkies, concoctions of sugar, hydrogenated fat and flavorings, replace meals. Ramen noodles, refined flour packed with flavorings and artificial flavor enhancers, provide a plastic wrapped hot snack for those whose only cooking skill lies in boiling water or turning on a microwave. Hamburgers, hot dogs, pizzas and other fast foods drive down the quality of farming and processing practice. Soft drinks replace other drinks, leading to large increases in sugar intake. The result is a dietary disaster area. Never have so many eaten so much fat and sugar.

How is it that a civilization that has brought so much progress in so many areas of human aspiration and idealism has let us down so badly in our most important activity – eating – and its equally important goal – health? It is easy to blame big business and agricultural pressure groups. But perhaps the real blame lies with us, with the casual, even careless approach we apply to how we grow and choose our food.

People who get a grip on their diet not only enjoy their food much more; they enjoy better health, happiness and longevity. It is terribly unfair that innocent children, born into modern, prosperous democratic societies – and too young to know any better – should be trapped in a vicious cycle of junk food addiction that will shorten their lives and make them forever dependent. How can we get it together to have food and diet worthy of the achievements of our civilization?

• The human species is facing evolutionary change. Two hundred years ago, the average height of a European shot up by 30 cm. Today the change is not upwards but outwards. In 1980, 50% of Americans were a healthy weight, 35% were overweight and "only" 15% were obese. Then the obesity boom took hold: by 2000 only 35% were healthy weight, 35% were overweight and 30% were obese.

FOOD PORN

chef-obsessed

Is gourmet cooking the new rock 'n' roll – or just an above-the-navel branch of pornography?

Network television offers more than 40 hours of food programming a week, and over the last five years the number of magazines about food and cooking doubled, their circulation tripled and readership quadrupled.

Fans of pornography argue that revelling in visual images of sex is a lot safer than all that messy business involving dating, seduction and bodily fluids. For the food porn fan, how much healthier must it be to let the eyes do the eating and avoid all that messy business with shopping, cooking and dealing with bodily fat issues? Besides, the real thing is never presented with such panache, perfect lighting, artistic arrangements, voyeuristic camera angles and sparkling voiceovers. As every food stylist knows, Vaseline plays a crucially important role, giving a glistening sheen to that lovingly photographed, glazed, maple-balsamic turkey breast.

The pioneer of food writing – as admired for her way with words as for her recipes themselves – was MFK Fisher. Her reputation was established during World War II with the austerity cookbook *How to Cook a Wolf* which famously included a recipe that began with the advice to borrow 50 cents to buy some hamburger meat and wilted vegetables. But

For the food porn fan, how much healthier to let the eyes do the eating?

Frances Kennedy Fisher had been profoundly influenced by her first hand experience of the food culture of Burgundy and regional France.

Her memories, woven into the tapestry of books such as *With Bold Knife and Fork* and *The Gastronomical Me*, helped a generation of aspiring cooks to move beyond the utilitarianism of food as fuel and learn to enjoy the sensuality of good flavors, artfully combined, then consumed in the convivial company of one's friends and family. Unusually for a food writer, she was elected to the American Academy of Arts and Letters. The James Beard Foundation's lifetime achievement award set the seal on her contribution. She wrote: "It seems to me that our three basic needs for food and security and

> Our needs for food and security and love are so mixed we can't think of one without the others

love are so mixed and mingled that we cannot straightly think of one without the others. So it happens that when I write about hunger I am really writing about love and the hunger for it. There is communion of more than our bodies when bread is broken and wine drunk."

In Britain it all started in 1960 with Elizabeth David. Her groundbreaking book *French Provincial Cooking* offered something new and exciting to Brits emerging from the shadow of post-war rationing. In her introduction she advocated *faites simple* – "keep it simple." But her three-page recipe for cassoulet (mastery of which was the *sine qua non* for marrying well in the 60s) was an Everest of complexity. She laid down the new ground rules for food, saying it should be "civilized without being over-civilized. That is to say, it has natural taste, smell, texture and much character. Often it looks beautiful, too. What it amounts to is that it is the rational, right and proper food for human beings to eat."

For the inspired cook the question arose: "Yeah, but A&P don't carry balsamic vinegar." Where could you find these desirable ingredients?

In the mid 1970s Georgio DeLuca, the proprietor of a cheese shop in the SoHo district of Manhattan, invited his friend Joel Dean to join him in founding a store that would "turn dinner into a creative exercise." That store, Dean & DeLuca, became a temple of the new cuisine and set a pattern that was visited and copied by retailers from around the US and the world. The very fact that it prospered reflected the new and aware food culture that was emerging.

The modern doyenne of food that is of impeccable provenance, fresh, local, organic and sympathetically prepared, is Alice Waters, whose Berkeley restaurant Chez Panisse is a pilgrimage destination and inspiration for foodies worldwide. Articles by Michael Pollan of the *New York Times* build awareness of food culture. His book, *The Botany of Desire*, explores the fundamental passions of food – sweetness (the story of the apple), abundance (the story of the potato) – as well as dealing with beauty and intoxication (tulips and marijuana), foods for the eye and the mind.

If cooking is the new rock 'n' roll then its Johnny Rotten must surely be Anthony Bourdain, whose confessional *Kitchen Confidential* is a warts-and-all description of drug-crazed kitchen antics that will give extra edge to those contemplating a fusion food menu.

When it comes to cooking at home, what with all those food magazines, cookbooks and TV shows to get through, a phone call to Domino's Pizza saves time and hassle. The convenience food market grew by 400% in the 1990s. Inevitably perhaps, the more we watch other people cook, the less we do it ourselves.

When we do cook, we rarely do so "from scratch," relying on prepared ingredients to ensure that everything goes to recipe once we get the apron on.

But behind it all is a growing appreciation that food is fun as well as fuel, that you can eat well and be well, that health and happiness are not

Health and happiness are not mutually exclusive at the table

mutually exclusive at the dinner table. "Gastro-porn" does indeed signal the emergence of a new food culture.

• Desirable urban apartments are now built with tiny, or no, kitchens. They offer little more than areas for a fridge and a microwave.

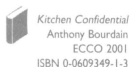

Kitchen Confidential
Anthony Bourdain
ECCO 2001
ISBN 0-0609349-1-3

EATING THE VIEW

a sense of awareness

You don't have to be an artist to appreciate beautiful countryside. Most of us are repelled by the sight of featureless expanses of barley and fields stripped of hedges, let alone covered by ugly buildings housing intensively reared farm animals.

In October 2001 Sandra Pepys, president of The British Society of Landscape Painters, organized an exhibition of landscape art at the Mall Galleries in London. All the artists

A typical CSA scheme involved members buying a share in a farm's output at the start of the season

represented agreed to give one third of their income from the show to The Council for the Protection of Rural England and the Soil Association, Britain's leading organic organization. Their offer acknowledged that the countryside they chose to paint often turned out to be under organic cultivation – a simple example of how individual actions count as a vote for both the kind of countryside consumers enjoy, and the food production practices they prefer. By literally "eating the view," the "man in the street" can support rural communities and initiatives.

Money circulates and the longer it can stay in a local area the more value it has. It is estimated that $10 spent in a supermarket on imported processed foods quickly finds its way out of the community and even out of the country. However, $10 spent on locally produced food has the economic impact of $28, as it changes hands several times before finding its way into the mainstream. Local producers earn a higher margin, saving on transport costs and benefiting from the added value of any processing they do

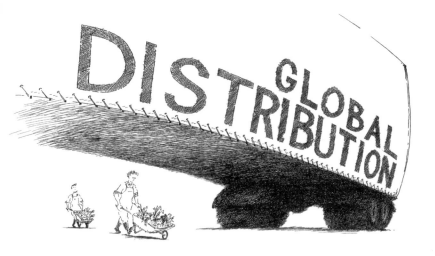

themselves. This supports the rural economy, without which much of the countryside would be little other than barren expanses of subsidized cereals.

Small farmers have latched onto direct selling and direct-to-consumer sales rose 37% from $592 million to $812 million between 1997 and 2002, according to USDA figures. These sales are now heading towards 1% of total US food sales.

Community Supported Agriculture (CSA) schemes and farmers' markets have been a key to bringing consumers into much closer links with the producers. A typical CSA scheme involves members of a community buying a share in a farm's output at the beginning of the season and then receiving weekly deliveries of produce. This guarantees fresh wholesome food for the shareholder and a secure source of income that enables efficient planning for the farmer. CSA farmers are more often women (40%), on average they're 10 years younger than the typical US farmer and many are newcomers to farming. Well over 90% operate to organic standards and more than 95% have a college education. Increasingly, as community involvement grows, these farms, though smaller than the average farm, become far more profitable per acre worked as they are selling direct to their customers with greatly reduced waste.

So, alternative retailing systems are flourishing, after a period when local retail business has been struggling – or closing. Supermarkets, in their turn, are responding and trying to meet the new demand for foods that have character

Supermarkets are trying to meet the new demand for foods that have character and local identity

and regional or local identity. The dead hand of centralized and intensive agriculture has held sway over the countryside for too many decades. Government, at last, recognizes that it is much easier to integrate its environmental, social and economic goals if it encourages "eat the view" practices.

The new "green consumerism" links wholesome food, beautiful countryside and sustainable agriculture. Entrepreneurialism may not come easily to farmers, but a new generation can thrive on such challenges. The average age of American farmers is 55 and rising, a sure sign of a declining industry. "Eating the view" can transform the countryside and the prospects of those who live in it while bringing fresh, wholesome and sustainably produced food to consumers. With lower food miles, less packaging and higher standards of animal welfare, "eating the view" is a win-win-win opportunity, and one that will encourage the move towards organic standards of production.

Bringing the Food Economy Home
Norberg-Hodge, Merrifield, Gorelick
Zed Books 2000
ISBN 1-5654914-6-7

www.nal.usda.gov/afsic/csa/

SLOW FOOD

taking time

The Slow Food movement started in Bra, a small town in the Piedmont region of Italy, at the foot of the Alps. It was prompted by the opening of a McDonald's restaurant in Rome in 1986 and adopted the slogan: "A firm defense of quiet material pleasure is the only way to oppose the universal folly of fast life."

Founded by Carlo Petrini, the Slow Food movement, with the snail as its symbol, focused initially on food and wine and produced a best-selling guide to Italian gastronomical treats.

But Petrini had a still greater vision – eco-gastronomy. "I want Slow Food not to be merely a gastronomical organization but [one that] deals with problems of the environment and world hunger without renouncing the right to pleasure," he said.

Perhaps as a reaction to its fast food culture, the US has seen rapid Slow Food growth. "The United States is natural Slow Food territory," says Petrini. "You have a huge move toward organic food and... microbreweries. Up until 10 or 20 years ago, you had two large companies [Busch and Miller] that dominated the beer market. Now you have 1,600 microbreweries." With more than 100 *convivia*, (local chapters) celebrating North American food traditions, Slow Food

A reaction to its fast food culture, the US has seen Slow Food growth

USA spans Cajun cuisine, organic traditions, heirloom vegetable and fruit varieties, farmhouse cheeses and other artisanal foods that have survived the industrialization of the fast food economy. A successful *Slow*

Food Guide to New York City – Restaurants, Markets and Bars has been followed by a similar guide covering Chicago. "Westward Slow!" in the Southwest and a "Field to Family" event in Iowa City show that this movement has spread far and wide.

Slow Food even has an office in Brussels, the EU capital. Here, they successfully protect many Italian producers from the complex administrative requirements that are impossible for small producers to comply with. When they set out to protect the Piedmontese cow, whose numbers were diminishing, Slow Food helped livestock producers to adopt

> The Slow Food Movement has led to Slow Cities, where the quality of the food is the foundation for an eco-gastronomic approach to life

organic and additive-free methods to produce a higher quality, lower fat beef. Market success came slowly, until Mad Cow Disease was discovered in Italian beef. Piedmontese beef quickly became every Italian's first choice.

Slow Food now has 65,000 members in 50 countries organized in 560 *convivia*. In the US alone there are over 62 chapters. Its *Salone del Gusto* "Taste Convention" is Italy's most popular food fair and draws international attention. Small food producers, "natural stewards of biodiversity," have discovered that shared ethical values can create global opportunities. Typical of these is Veli Galas, a Turkish beekeeper. He won the Slow Food Award for a honey made in the trunks of trees in a forest near the Black Sea.

The Slow Food Movement has led to Slow Cities, where the quality of food is the foundation for a cultural, environmental and "eco-gastronomic" approach to urban life. Over 30 Italian towns are now members. Though none has yet earned the coveted "Cittaslow" snail logo, it is hoped that cities and towns worldwide will move toward attaining Slow City status and set an example of how urban living can satisfy "neo-humanist" aspirations. Many participating towns have already seen economic growth. *Newsweek* magazine even suggested that Slow Food and Cittaslow were a unique, Italian response to globalization.

Key requirements to become a Slow
City include:

- Encouraging good food with farmers'
  markets, traditional cuisine, organic
  agriculture and no genetically
  modified products.
- Prohibiting car alarms, TV aerials,
  advertising billboards and neon signs.
- Ecological transport with cycle
  paths, expanded pedestrian areas
  and limits on cars.
- Tree planting, recycling and new parks.
- Urging businesses, schools and
  government offices to adjust hours
  to enable people to enjoy a slow
  midday meal with family and friends.

- Slow Food sees children as the Slow
Foodies of the future and seeks to
educate them in the taste of food and in
how it is produced. They even produce
a book teaching kids about flavor and its
appreciation through "aware" tasting.

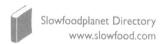

Slowfoodplanet Directory
www.slowfood.com

MACROBIOTICS

healthy eating – healthy living

Definition:
1. "great life," in both length and quality;
2. the seeker after health and longevity.

Macrobiotics was the only wholefood/healthy eating message of the 1960s and '70s, inspiring the natural foods and organic movement. The first natural food stores that appeared in the '70s in the US and Europe stuck to macrobiotic

> Health is not just the absense of disease but good appetite, good humor and clarity of thinking

principles, selling grains and legumes and organic vegetables and avoiding processed foods, especially any containing sugar.

Macrobiotic medicine mirrors elements of traditional Japanese folk medicine but puts primary emphasis on diet. *Zen Macrobiotics* by George Ohsawa was the original guide to macrobiotic living. In it he describes positive health. "Health is not just the absence of disease but is defined in positive terms as: No fatigue, good appetite, deep and good sleep, good memory, good humor, clarity of thinking and doing and, most importantly, gratitude. The four-part way to achieve this is set out as: Natural food, no medicine, no surgery, no inactivity."

Macrobiotic directions for a natural food diet are:
• No industrialized food and drink such as sugar, soft drinks, dyed food, canned or bottled food.
• Wholegrains and vegetables as the core of the diet with animal products eaten in smaller amounts or not at all. When Ohsawa wrote there was no organic

meat sector, so he proposed occasional game and fish.

- Food should be produced without chemical fertilizers and pesticides, i.e organic food.
- Avoid food that comes from a long distance.
- Choose foods in season – eating in season harmonizes with the body's natural seasonal changes. (It also ensures freshness and avoids preservatives.)
- Avoid nightshade plants: eggplant, potato, tomato – they contain toxic solanine alkaloids.
- No chemical seasonings (i.e. MSG), coloring or preservatives.
- No coffee, although tea is allowed.
- Yeasted foods kept to a minimum – natural leaven preferred.
- Chew every mouthful 50 times or more.
- Low liquid intake – Ohsawa argued that kidney function did not need large amounts of water.

Some of these may seem excessive, but it was macrobiotics that introduced us to the "brown rice and lentils" of the alternative lifestyle. A diet high in wholegrains, legumes and vegetables was certainly cheaper than a diet based on processed foods, animal products and imported luxuries, but it was its health benefits that spurred devotees on.

The Taoist principle of complementary opposites, Yin and Yang, underpins macrobiotic theory. Some foods are more yang, others more yin. A food's characteristics, when consumed, translates into a similar yin-yang balance in the consumer. In this way, if one is overexcited and energetic (excess yang) one can eat more bland yin foods to reach a less stressed state – cabbage, carrots, milk, pears

If you eat the right foods, a healthy body will extract what it needs

and potatoes. If one is tired and dreamy (excess yin) one can energize and focus by choosing more rich and hot yang foods – beef, chicken, eggs, peanuts, peppers and onions. Success in macrobiotics comes when you find a healthy equilibrium and then instinctively choose the foods that maintain it.

The concept of "biological transmutation" infuses macrobiotics, the idea that the digestive system can create nutrients that are not already in the food you eat. It argues that if you eat the right foods, a healthy body will extract the balance of nutrients that it needs, manufacturing them if necessary with the help of the gut flora or by other processes.

Many macrobiotic-dieters, however, stuck too rigidly to the rules, with poor results.

Many macrobiotic-dieters stuck too rigidly to the rules

Ohsawa advised against such rigidity, arguing that the healthy constitution achieved through macrobiotics confers the ability to relax the rules sometimes with no ill effect.

Good health is one aspect of macrobiotic living. On a broader level, macrobiotics also aspires to a central role in bringing about social evolution and global stability. Ohsawa even saw world peace as the eventual successful outcome of the universal practice of macrobiotics.

The "win-win" equation runs: healthy food = healthy people = healthy societies = peace. Ohsawa died in 1966, just a few months before the Peace Olympics which he had planned. One of his colleagues, Michio Kushi, went on to found East-West macrobiotic study centers around the world and the movement is still active and growing. The core ideas of macrobiotics had also entered the mainstream. Back in 1966 Dr. Fredrick Stare, the eminent Harvard nutritionist, wrote in *Reader's Digest:* "Macrobiotics is the diet that's killing our kids," so alarmed was he at its departure from convention. Today the Harvard School of Public Health, led by Walter Willett, the Frederick John Stare Professor of Epidemiology and Nutrition, cites macrobiotics as an example of the kind of diet that Americans should adopt to avoid diet-related health disease and excess body weight.

• Ohsawa urged macrobiotic-followers to read *Erewhon*, the novel by Samuel Butler, describing a Utopia in which sick people are thrown in prisons and criminals treated in hospitals. In 1974 a Pennsylvania prison initiated a program of macrobiotic food for prisoners. Rates of violence fell, as did the number of re-offenses.

Macrobiotics for Beginners
Jo Sandifer, Bob Lloyd
Piatkus 2000
ISBN 0-7499211-9-6

SOIL AND SOLUTIONS

why did we go chemical?

Way back in 1836, with the science of chemistry in its infancy, one food technologist, Baron Justus von Liebig, took a look at what made plants grow and what made food taste good. He worked out that the key elements in soil that nourished plants were nitrogen, phosphorus and potassium and decided to "improve" soil by synthesizing these ingredients himself. This was the start of "modern" farming.

His ideas didn't catch on, the chemicals cost money and, although in the short term crop yields improved, farmers found that they needed more and more chemicals in order to maintain yields. The economics simply didn't work. By 1863, when Liebig was 65 years old, he was disillusioned with his attempts to help farming, and wrote: "I have sinned against the Creator and, justly, I have been punished. I wanted to improve His work because, in my blindness, I believed that a link in the astonishing chain of laws that govern and constantly renew life on the surface of the Earth had been forgotten. It seemed to me that weak and insignificant man had to redress this oversight."

Notwithstanding his recantation, chemicals continued to play a part in agriculture – as a short-term fix to build up soil fertility and as part of the curriculum at agricultural colleges. Meanwhile, the American prairies, a vast, unexploited reservoir of fertility, were opened up to farming, and European agriculture had to struggle against cheap imports of American wheat and beef.

However, by the 1930s the soil fertility of the American Midwest was so exhausted that the Dust Bowl had become a devastating reality. The humus-exhausted topsoil, no longer held together by organic matter, simply blew away. This event shocked farmers around the world and the organic movement was born.

A study of Chinese, Korean and Japanese agriculture, *Farmers of Forty Centuries* by F. H. King (1911), showed how farmers had increased the fertility of their farmland by returning organic matter to the soil. Around the same time Sir Albert Howard, in India to teach

World War II showed the need for agricultural self-sufficiency

modern agricultural methods, soon realized that he had more to learn than to teach. He was the father of modern composting, bringing the "Indore Process" back to Britain, where it was enthusiastically adopted by many British farmers. Among these was Lady Eve Balfour who used it at her farm in Haughley, Suffolk. She went on to found the Soil Association, the founding organization of the global organic movement, in 1946. In Pennsylvania, in 1947, J.I. Rodale founded the Soil and Health Foundation, subsequently known as the Rodale Institute. Rodale coined the term "organic," which came to describe what was previously known as

"permanent farming" i.e. farming that could be sustained forever without exhausting the land.

The Second World War showed the need for agricultural self-sufficiency. It also led to tremendous growth in the production of nitrogen-based explosives and toxic organophosphorous chemicals which were developed as potential nerve gas weaponry. After World War II the manufacturers of explosives and nerve gas found themselves with huge overcapacity. As debates raged about the future direction of agriculture, ICI in Britain lobbied heavily for the wider use of agrichemicals. It needed to divert its production capacity from a war on the Axis powers to a war on Nature, using nitrates and pesticides as the primary weapons. The Soil Association proposed a continuation of wartime quasi-organic methods and argued that healthy soils were needed to produce healthy plants and animals if humans themselves were to enjoy good health. Farmers were cautious about adopting agrichemicals as they knew only too well the dangers of exhausting fertility and becoming dependent on artificial fertilizers. In the US crop-specific subsidies to farmers discouraged crop rotation and led to increased use of fertilizers and pesticides. The absence of nitrate fertilizers during the war had shown how depleted of fertility American soils had become.

While increased yields became the norm, soil structure, fertility and health declined further and plants became more prone to insect and fungal attack. Weeds also grew rapidly when fertilizers were applied, so herbicide use boomed. All these chemicals inevitably damaged the environment.

But by now farmers, or at least their land, were addicted to chemicals. Overproduction led to surpluses, which were dumped on developing countries, damaging the livelihoods of small farmers, many of whom were driven out of business and forced to migrate to urban centers. Here aid kept them alive, while they sought work as cheap labor or migrated to Europe or North America to look for work.

The organic movement looked stymied. For as long as governments subsidized overproduction, farmers would use artificial fertilizers in preference to natural methods. Consider, for example, that there have never been subsidies for a field of clover, even though it increases the nitrogen and the humus content of the soil. But a core of organic farmers soldiered on, committed to doing right by the land and by nature. By the 1960s a market for their products was emerging among consumers who did not want pesticide residues in their food or to see the countryside ruined. That market continues to grow today.

• In 1974, the Soil Association produced the world's first written standards that defined exactly what food production qualified as organic.

• Globally, the market for organic food now exceeds $25 billion, with the United States ($10.5b), Germany ($3b) and Britain ($1.5b), the countries where agrochemicals had once been most enthusiastically adopted, showing the fastest growth. The concepts of "permanent" or "sustainable" farming are evolving further into the idea of "regenerative" farming, embodying the idea of creating even better land than we started out with. With modern organic farming methods, that's a realistic goal.

The Organic Tradition
Philip Conford (editor)
Green Books 1988
ISBN 1-8700980-9-9

WHY ORGANICS?

why destroy the planet?

Why do so many producers, consumers and policymakers see "organics" as a desirable alternative to conventional farming? Well, the arguments for organics are powerful: food safety and quality, sustainability, environment, employment, rural economy and animal welfare.

Food Safety and Quality
Most organic consumers seek, above all, to avoid pesticides. The traceability required

Organic crops have higher levels of Vitamin C, magnesium, iron and phosphorus

for all certified organic food ensures strict standards for growing and processing. Excluded are pesticides, processing chemicals, genetically modified organisms (GMOs), hydrogenated fats, phosphoric acid, artificial colorings, preservatives, artificial sweeteners and flavor enhancers, hormones and antibiotics. Not everyone cares about all these things, but only organic food offers a comprehensive guarantee of their absence – backed up by an international inspection and certification system. Although organic rules allow white sugar, white flour, alcohol (there's even organic rum) and other foods that are not really "healthy," organic food appeals to the health-conscious (those who eat more vegetables, fruit and fiber and less fat and sugar).

In April 2001, The Worthington Study reviewed 41 other studies carried out on crops grown using organic matter or inorganic fertilizers. In all cases the organic crops had higher levels of Vitamin C (27% more), magnesium (29%), iron (21%) and phosphorus (14%).

Sustainability

Organic farming began with concerns about the loss of topsoil, disappearing forests and the risk that we could run out of land to feed ourselves. Fossil fuels and carbon output are extra concerns.

To rebuild topsoil, organic farmers plant green manures, make compost and undersow crops with clover to increase organic matter (humus) in soil. The result is better water retention and soil fertility. Conventional agriculture loses arable land every year. One cause is salination: chemical fertilizers destroy humus so that frequent irrigation is needed, water retention is minimal and salts build up. This can't be sustained. Building humus also captures and stores carbon, thus reducing global warming. Organic farmers who plough only occasionally and use green manures can accumulate more than 800 pounds of carbon per acre per year. Organic farming also uses less fossil fuel, preferring human labor to heavy machinery. Fertilizers and pesticides are made from fossil fuels, too; organic farmers use less of them.

The arithmetic of farming can appear ludicrous: it takes 12 calories of fossil fuels to produce one calorie of food grain in industrial agriculture. Organic farming uses five calories. (An African peasant with a hoe uses 1 calorie of energy to produce 20 calories of food). Organic arable production can be 35% more energy efficient, and organic dairy production 74% more efficient than non-organic production. Worldwide, farmers now use 10 times more fertilizer and spend 17 times more on pesticides than in 1950. The share of the harvest lost to pests, however, is unchanged.

The Environment

Organic farms generally support higher levels of wildlife. 40% more birds were found in a three-year UK study of 44 farms, twice as many butterflies and five times as many wild arable plants.

Further, no nitrate fertilizer is used on organic farms and there are limits on manure use; so nitrate pollution of water is low. Excess nitrate runoff causes algae growth that de-oxygenates water, killing fish and aquatic plants.

Employment

The use of pesticides, herbicides, chemical fertilizers, intensive animal rearing systems and the creation of bigger fields mean fewer workers. So, rural employment declines and poverty among farmers increases. Of the 1.2 billion people who earn less than one dollar a day, 800 million live in rural areas. In the US in 1950, half of the money spent on food found its way to the farmer. The figure today is just 7%. The difference goes to processors, chemical companies, machinery suppliers and agribusiness cartels. Research on 200 organic projects in the developing world showed that conventional yields could increase by 93% – and more. Employment and soil fertility also increase.

Rural Economy

As government policies force farm laborers off the land, the rural economy declines. Money earned and spent locally circulates several times and supports rural communities. A farmer who buys in chemicals and machinery, and ships out products, has little effect on the local economy. Many Midwestern states in the US are now suffering rural depopulation and some farm families are now dependent on food donations.

Animal Welfare

Organic standards for animal care are strict. In 2002 Compassion in World Farming compared the standards for organic farms against 15 criteria for animal welfare. Organic farming achieved between 11 and 14 out of 15 for five different livestock groups. Conventional systems scored between four and seven. Much of the growth in the sale of organics has come from vegetarians, many of whom have converted to eating organic meat because they approve of the animal welfare standards.

People often choose organic food for specific reasons – avoidance of a particular pesticide such as lindane, or horror at the cruelties inflicted on battery hens. However, as the whole range of issues is further understood, the commitment to eating organically deepens.

• About 5,000,000,000 acres of soil have been degraded through human activities – that's 15% of the Earth's land area, an area larger than the US and Mexico combined.

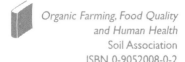

Organic Farming, Food Quality and Human Health
Soil Association
ISBN 0-9052008-0-2

SUBSIDIES USA

who gains, who loses?

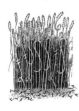

Subsidies keep less healthy foods such as hamburgers, soft drinks and hydrogenated fat cheap and thus encourage obesity by distorting people's food choices. But their real victims are smaller family farms and the global economy. Real hardship and poverty are caused, worldwide, by the subsidy system of the US and EU. Rich countries' subsidies to their own farmers amount to seven times their annual foreign aid of $50 billion. Along with protectionist import barriers they prevent those poor countries' farmers from selling their products to the rich world.

So how do subsidies cause poverty?

1. Cheap exports of subsidized surplus food undermine local agricultural economies; farmers cannot compete with subsidized grain and meat.

2. World prices for all food are kept artificially low by subsidies. This is the main cause of poverty among the 1.2 billion farmers worldwide who earn less than $1 per day. Although cheap food prices help those on low incomes, the urban poor should not be used as an excuse for keeping the rural poor in poverty. It is rural poverty that fuels the exodus to the urban slums fuelling the growth of numbers of urban poor. The foundation of developing country economies is agriculture,

World prices for all food are kept artificially low by subsidies

usually 50% to 80% of gross national product (GNP) compared to 1% of US or UK GNP. So if farmers do well, the whole economy thrives. The more farmers earn, the more they spend on material goods and, crucially, the more they spend on educating their kids, giving them the opportunity of better jobs and better incomes.

3. Subsidies also drive small farmers in the US and EU countries out of business. They support large farms that practice environmentally damaging monoculture. The income of farmers is set by the government; if they go bankrupt it is because of policy decisions, not market forces.

Cheap Exports

Farm policy in the US and EU involves buying the farmers' surpluses and storing them. These are then dumped as "aid" or sold cheap to developing countries. Some surpluses are

Subsidies drive small farmers out of business and support damaging monoculture farming

converted into meat and dairy products that are then exported or given away – a convenient disposal route.

In Mexico, where subsidized American corn is imported under the North American Free Trade Agreement (NAFTA), 15 million people will lose their livelihoods. If there were no US subsidies Mexican farmers could profitably export corn to the US. In the dry Sahel countries of Africa, small farmers cannot compete with EU dumping of surplus subsidized cereals and so move to the cities in search of work. The land is left to pastoral nomads whose animals graze away what little vegetation there is, increasing desertification.

World Food Price Distortion

It is the Chicago Board of Trade that sets low prices for agricultural commodities: pork bellies, beef, corn, soybeans, wheat and soybean oil. These prices then become the yardstick for world pricing. It might be called a "market," but prices are the direct result of government subsidy policy rather than of market laws of supply and demand. All this influence – and the US has only 8% of the world's farmland!

The average American farm now earns half its income from government subsidies, but the level of subsidy to corn and soybean farmers is higher still – nearly 100%. Without subsidies, prices would have to double and the income of all the world's food producers would increase dramatically.

EXAMPLE

A farmer in Kenya grows maize at a cost of 4.5 cents per pound, which is more than the US "market" price of 3.5 cents per pound. But the true cost of production to an American farmer is 6 cents per pound. In this Alice in Wonderland world, the more efficient Kenyan farmer can't compete with the less efficient American farmer who has the mighty American taxpayer subsidizing their artificially reduced farm-gate price.

If the Chicago price was unsubsidized, it would go up; the Kenyan farmer could compete and become more profitable. He would be able to pay for healthcare, education and manufactured goods – all to the benefit and future stability of Kenya. Instead, if the Kenyan farmer tries to sell for five cents per pound, in an attempt to make a profit, grain traders will import the cheaper American corn (cheaper even with freight costs).

Emigration, war, refugees and shantytowns are the result of agricultural communities collapsing. The lucky ones get a job in Europe or the USA, often illegally and in exploitative conditions; quite often – ironically – in agriculture. They then send their earnings home, to support their families who have stayed behind on the land. It is a wasteful and inefficient way of allocating the world's human and agricultural resources.

Harm to American and European small farmers

Family farmers, including organic farmers, receive lower levels of subsidy. Without subsidies big

Kenyan farmers can't compete with US farmers subsidized by taxpayers

farmers would profit less from planting prairies of corn and soybeans or intensifying animal production. Small-scale farming would stage a comeback. Food prices might go up a little, but probably no more than the $30 per week per household that subsidies cost the average American family. The USDA spends much of its annual budget on storage and warehousing costs for surpluses, administration costs and fraud control. Further billions are spent subsidizing the conversion of surpluses into sugar and "bio-fuels." A child could see the waste in this.

So who gains from subsidies?

• Big farming corporations do. **The subsidy**

system encourages "monoculture," mainly of feed crops. The large, heavily mechanized agri-businesses, the biggest users of chemical fertilizers, pesticides and herbicides, get the biggest slice of the subsidy pie.

• Agrichemical manufacturers. Sales would be lower if small family farms prevailed, since they use fewer chemicals.

• Intensive chicken, beef and pork producers. The growth of the cheap meat industry is linked to the growth of the fast-food industry which depends on subsidized animal feed. Without it meat would cost generally more and

Most aid to developing countries is aimed at increasing their reliance on hybrid seeds and agrichemicals

hamburgers would cost 2-3 times as much as they do. Subsidized burgers and chicken nuggets come at an awful cost.

Subsidies vs Aid

After military aid, most aid to developing countries is agricultural. Much of it is aimed at increasing – yes, increasing – their reliance on hybrid seeds, agrichemicals and machinery. Recently it has been targeted at supporting the export of genetically engineered biotechnology products. All of these have long-term effects on yields, soil fertility and the rural economy.

The repayment of Third World debt results in a net transfer of resources from struggling South to prosperous North. In 1998, Third World Countries put about $114.6 billion into the private and public coffers of the North. The 41 poorest countries paid $1.7 billion more than they received in aid. Since 1981, the South has transferred to the North $3.7 trillion, and yet today more that $200 billion is still owed. Many countries have to borrow even more in order to repay interest and debt. Governments in the South have had to sacrifice their internal economies, abandon health care, education, employment, popular housing, land demarcation for indigenous peoples, agrarian reform and environmental protection in order to keep up payments. Natural resources have been squandered in the attempt to keep up interest payments. Most of the burden of repayment falls on agriculture, an agriculture struggling to survive already against the pressure of prices depressed by US and European subsidies.

Given the chance, farmers could compete internationally. Third World farmers as well as US and EU family farmers would benefit economically. Disease, overpopulation and poverty would be alleviated by increased domestic and foreign income. The annual income benefit for the developing world could be as much as $1.75 trillion if food prices found their natural unsubsidized level.

In 2004, the WTO agreed with a complaint against US cotton subsidies, which drive the price of cotton down to 28¢. The cost of production to a Texas farmer is around 75¢, and he profits, because the subsidy more than makes up the difference. The cost of production to a West African farmer is around 35¢ – he loses money growing cotton and goes out of business.

State of the World 2002
W.W. Norton + Company 2002
ISBN 0-3930505-3-X

THE DIGESTIVE SYSTEM

chewing it over

The food we eat contains protein, carbohydrates, fats, vitamins and minerals. It also contains other elements that nourish us in ways that are, as yet, not completely understood. If different people eat the same foods some will gain the nutrients they need, other will experience nutrient deficiencies. Why?

We need to look first at the "soil food web." A plant sends its roots into the soil in search

An organic farmer needs to do a lot of composting to build up a new soil food web

of nutrients as food. In healthy soil there are some 500 known organisms and it is these that provide the nutrients. Plants produce

"exudates," which include sugars that nourish and regulate the balance of life around its root system – while attracting micro-organisms. Other micro-organisms are food for other life forms whose excrement provides plant nutrients. A complex symbiosis exists. It's a plant's "mycorrhizae," or "fungus-roots," that ensure this close mutually beneficial relationship between soil and plant roots. Thin white mycorrhizal fungal filaments extend the "reach" of the roots and enable them to draw nutrients from the furthest parts of the soil. The use of pesticides, fungicides or herbicides devastates soil organism populations. So do nitrate fertilizers, but they compensate by providing concentrated, readily available nutrients direct to the roots. This is why a "chemical" farmer can adopt chemical use overnight but an organic farmer needs to do a lot of composting to build up a new soil food web.

So what about digestion? The food we eat is converted into what the Chinese politely call "night soil" – produced while we sleep and our digestive system works away. It is so similar to soil that many parasitic worms can thrive as well in our intestines as in the soil.

Over 500 different organisms – "intestinal flora" – have been identified in our digestive system, weighing a total of 6 lbs. The human body also has "roots" that function in the same way as a plant's roots, delivering nutrients from the "soil" in the intestines to the rest of the body. These are the intestinal "villi" – root-like protruberances that pack the small intestine.

The villi are protected from direct contact with food by a layer of mucus composed of intestinal flora, *Lactobacillus acidophilus* in particular. If this protective layer is eroded, the villi, packed with tiny capillaries, bleed and are unable to absorb the nutrients that the body needs from the liquefied food. It is intestinal bacteria, such as *Acidophilus*, that carry nutrients to the villi and create others such as B vitamins. They also control undesirable bacteria by secreting natural antibiotics. This is the human "digestive food web" that has evolved to enable us to exist on a wide variety of foods.

However, there are quite a few ways this can go wrong, and they echo the way that the soil food web can be upset by nitrate fertilizers, pesticides and fungicides.

Eating sugar and white flour products encourages yeasts to grow and compete with

Over 50 different organisms exist in the human digestive system

the *Acidophilus* bacteria. Yeasts irritate the villi, creating gases and causing bloating and cramping. The villi are exposed to nutrients that have not been filtered by the layer of flora and absorb unwanted substances that the body must excrete, a condition known as "malabsorption syndrome." Antibiotic use eradicates large numbers of intestinal flora, in the same way that fungicides eradicate mycorrhizal fungi. Stress can have a physical effect; the intestines twist with "anxiety" and internal rubbing removes patches of flora. Other flora-harming substances include alcohol, chlorine in drinking water, cigarettes and preservatives. Milk can cause harm, particularly in lactose-intolerant people.

Maintaining a healthy digestive food web means introducing the same conditions that composting provides to create a healthy soil food web: plenty of organic matter (by consuming leafy vegetables and wholegrains), inoculation with the "right" bacteria (by eating yogurt, sauerkraut or sourdough bread),

It is extraordinary that with all our scientific knowledge we allow ourselves to eat so badly

careful chewing to ensure small particle sizes, avoidance of substances that harm the desirable bacteria that make up the intestinal flora. Then the "soil" of the mucus membrane and the "microbial lawn" of the organisms that dwell in it can work at optimal levels of effectiveness.

It is extraordinary that, with all our scientific knowledge of nutrition and the human body, we should – millions of us – allow ourselves to be persuaded to eat so badly.

• "As above, so below." Eating organically requires the same understanding and harnessing of natural processes that farming organically requires. Success comes from achieving a healthy bacterial community and in preventing the "dysbiosis," or system, failure that leads to disease.

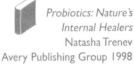

Probiotics: Nature's Internal Healers
Natasha Trenev
Avery Publishing Group 1998
ISBN 0-8952984-7-3

http://pleosanum.com/newspdf/may2004.pdf

OBESITY

dieting can make you fat

"I have more flesh than another man, and therefore more frailty."
Falstaff, Henry IV: Part One, Shakespeare

If school children were injected with a disease that crippled them, shortened their lifespan and increased their dependency on health services there would be outrage. Yet we watch, helpless, as a combination of heavily advertized junk food and inactivity achieves a similar result through obesity – a condition that is rarely curable.

Children's TV programs are the main promoters of foods such as sugary breakfast cereals, candy, soft drinks and fast food. It is left to "pester power" to do the rest. If obesity doesn't strike in childhood, modern lifestyles make it a risk at all stages of life. Eating too many calories is half the problem; not burning them off is the other half. Watching television,

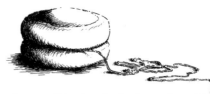

using cars, living in suburbs that make walking or cycling impractical all combine to reduce calorie usage. So, food is not the only culprit, but it is a major factor.

America claims world leadership in obesity. Fat is epidemic, with an estimated 65% of Americans overweight, of whom 30%

An estimated 65% of Americans are overweight

are obese. The problem is even more pronounced among the poor, especially African-Americans.

Obesity is responsible for 325,000 American deaths annually, more than motor vehicles, illegal drugs, alcohol and firearms combined. Overweight people are more likely than others to die from heart disease, stroke, kidney failure, gallstones, arthritis, pregnancy complications and depression. It is set to overtake smoking in the US as the leading cause of death, and it kills eight times more than die of AIDS.

Beyond the human costs, the financial costs of obesity are staggering: some $117 billion annually in healthcare and lost wages in the

> The financial costs of obesity are staggering: some $117 billion annually in healthcare and lost wages in the US alone

US. The "five-a-day" campaign to encourage Americans to eat more fruit and vegetables spends $2 million a year in promotion. McDonald's spends more than $1 billion and Coca-Cola spends $800 million on advertising. Exactly how much encouragement do we need to become obese?

The lawyers who successfully sued "Big Tobacco" are now suing the fast food and snack industries – known collectively as "Big Fat." These companies, the lawyers say, use manipulative strategies to market unhealthy products that, eaten regularly, can lead to disease and death. Concerned nutritionists have called for a "fat tax" on such food.

So what about dieting? Slimming is rarely successful, even in the short term. If you reduce food intake the rate at which your metabolism burns calories slows down – a natural survival mechanism inherited from our ancestors, whose food supply was uncertain. When you start eating normally again, calories are burned off more slowly and weight accumulates. This "yo-yo dieting" can lead to net weight gain. Regular exercise helps reduce weight, but obesity makes exertion difficult. Choosing the right foods can help: foods that are high in complex carbohydrates (starch) and fiber help to create the feeling of fullness that stops you overeating and so reduces your calorie intake.

What about non-nutritive, artificial foods that replace sugar and fat? Users of the sweetener Aspartame often complain that using it in place of sugar overrides that sense of "fullness," tempting those who eat "diet" foods actually to eat more. Similar negative effects can be found with artificial fats, such as Olestra. These have been cleverly developed to escape digestion but the side effect of "anal leakage" means they are not a success with consumers.

Dr. Paula Baillie-Hamilton, who holds a doctorate in human metabolism from Oxford University, has noted that in the 1960s, before hormones and antibiotic growth promoters came into wider use, organophosphates (insecticide) were used to promote animal weight gain. They slow down the metabolism, reduce the desire to exercise and thereby increase fat accumulation. Organo-phosphate residue is of the most common pesticides found in food.

Body Mass Index (BMI)
How to calculate:

$$\frac{\text{Body weight in pounds}}{(\text{height in inches}) \times (\text{height in inches})} \times 703 = BMI$$

Over 25 BMI = Overweight
Over 30 BMI = Obese

EXAMPLE
For example, a person who is 6'3" and weighs 220 pounds has a body mass index of 27.5 – overweight.

$$\frac{220 \text{ pounds}}{(75 \times 75)} \times 703 = 27.5$$

BMI calculators can be found at:

www.cdc.gov/nccdphp/dnpa/bmi/calc-bmi.htm

www.consumer.gov/weightloss/bmi.htm

VERY FAST FOOD

and the very slow people it creates

*"Those who do not have enough
time for good health will not have good
health for enough time."*
Paul Bragg

Americans are getting fat. On any day, one in every four Americans visits a fast food restaurant. The growth of the market for fast food is spectacular – in the US it has gone from $6 billion in 1970 to $110 billion in 2000, nearly 20 times growth. Having saturated the market in the US and Europe, McDonald's is opening branches in China. They now have 28,700 outlets in 120 countries. The startling figures don't just relate to beef, though; consumption of french fries has increased from 4 pounds to 30 pounds per person per year, all cooked in beef tallow or hydrogenated fat (see chapter "Vegetarians – Eating With Conscience"). The soft drinks that are packaged in the "meal deals" of fast food outlets ensure that a good dose of sugar is consumed with every burger and fries.

Obesity rates have, inevitably, rocketed in line with fast food production. The $320 billion cost of obesity to society is twice the income of the fast food industry. Fast food isn't the only cause of obesity, but the high levels of fat and sugar in a fast food meal are many times greater than those found in home-cooked food or in conventional restaurant food. Levels of dietary fiber and vegetables are much lower. The combination undermines all the health advice of government and nutritional bodies.

Some nutritionists call for a tax on fast food to reduce consumption and also to help pay for the cost of the obesity and illness that fast food generates. Yet government policy operates in the opposite direction. Their main effect is to keep the price of animal feed, sugar and fats such as rapeseed and soy oil unnaturally cheap. These are the key ingredients of fast food. Take away the subsidies and a burger, cola and fries meal priced at $2.49 would cost $7.50. Cattle feed costs in the US are lower today than they were in 1933, during severe economic depression. Low feed costs, the use of hormones and antibiotics as growth promoters, "market deficiency" payments, cheap immigrant labor, intensive rearing conditions and special tax breaks all work to keep the cost of a fast food meal extremely low and yet very profitable. No similar basket of payments exists for producers of vegetables or other nutritionally desirable foods. If a fast food meal was priced at its true cost and penalized for its health costs to society, then we would see a very different picture. Meanwhile, the industry is praised as an example of popular capitalism while being heavily dependent on state support.

The shiny presentation of fast food restaurants belies another problem: the unsanitary conditions on intensive factory farms that has led to a flurry of food borne diseases such as *E.coli*, *Salmonella* and *Campylobacter*. Food poisoning cases in the UK have risen from fewer than 19,000 in 1989 to more than 100,000 in 1999. *E.coli* has long been a problem, caused by the fecal contamination of beef in the slaughterhouse. Symptoms of contamination are stomach cramps and diarrhea. However, in 1983 a new, mutated and highly toxic form of the bacteria emerged, *E.coli* O157:H7. Its symptoms include death (200 per year in the US) and kidney failure (see chapter "Deadly Diseases"). The emergence of this new, deadly form of *E.coli* coincides with the introduction of intensive feedlot rearing of beef, dependent on continuous feeding of antibiotics. In Britain the feeding of animal remains to livestock was banned in 1996 as a result of the BSE epidemic among cattle and the risk that it was linked to variant Creutzfeld Jacobs Disease (CJD) among humans. In the US the feeding of sheep, cow, dog

US cattle are fed the remains of certain dead animals

and cat remains to cattle was banned in 1997. Yet there are no prohibitions on feeding dead chickens, pigs or horses, or even cattle blood. Cattle remains may be fed to chickens. Chicken manure may be fed to cattle. With practices like these, the spread of disease is inevitable and high-speed slaughterhouse practices, where "gut table" spillages are commonplace, only increase the risk of contamination further.

"Avian flu" – a virulent flu virus infecting chickens via fecal contamination – led to the slaughter of millions of infected chickens in early 2004. Previously harmless to humans, it has mutated to be fatal to humans – health authorities fear it may mutate to be transmitted from human to human, causing a global pandemic.

The situation is now so dire that we are seeing lawsuits organized by the lawyers who successfully sued tobacco companies. The legal principle, that a manufacturer has a duty to warn consumers of the dangers of their product, has been established. Where will it end and to what extent will government intervene to control this run-away industry?

• One of the largest beneficiaries of US government subsidies is Archer Daniels Midland (ADM), a leading processor of animal products and supplier of ingredients to the fast-food industry. In a secretly recorded conversation the president of the company commented, at a price-fixing meeting with Japanese executives: "Our competitors are our friends, our customers are our enemies." The vice-chairman of ADM was sent to prison in 1999 for price-fixing on lysine (a chicken feed additive made from subsidized corn). This was after they had been fined heavily for fixing prices on corn syrup, an essential sweetener in the US. It is, of course, subsidized, as is the corn from which it is made.

• In the UK an estimated 5.5 million people a year are affected by food poisoning. Of those, 71% believed their food-borne illness was caused as a result of eating in a restaurant, cafe or fast food outlet.

• More than 1 billion adults worldwide are affected by obesity with 500,000 people in the US and Western Europe dying from obesity-related diseases each year.

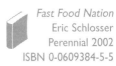

Fast Food Nation
Eric Schlosser
Perennial 2002
ISBN 0-0609384-5-5

INTENSIVE AGRICULTURE

how intense can you get?

One hundred thousand years ago the Earth lived on its natural wealth: rich soils produced food for plants that fed animals that fed predators. The hunting to extinction of large mammals was the first step towards the loss of the Earth's resources. Domestication of grazing animals and the use of fire led to the destruction of forests and creation of pasture.

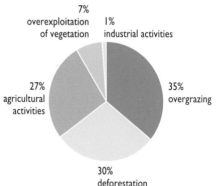

7%
overexploitation
of vegetation

1%
industrial activities

27%
agricultural
activities

35%
overgrazing

30%
deforestation

Agriculture followed, giving rise to the growth of civilizations, beginning in Sumer in the Tigris-Euphrates river system. Sumer's richly productive irrigated land, however, eventually became saline and eroded. Over a span of 2,500 years the world's first culture rose, flourished and then disappeared from history. In our own time, the last 50 years in the US has seen 55 million acres lost to salination. The "heartland" states, where intensified industrial agriculture dominates, are losing 5 to10 tons of topsoil per acre each year.

Such an outcome is brought on by the "cascade effect" of agricultural deterioration; all of which starts with nitrates, the key chemical fertilizer.

In the cascade effect:
• nitrates wipe out nitrogen-fixing bacteria in soil and encourage bacteria that break down organic matter and humus.

- loss of humus leads to reduced water retention, meaning more irrigation is needed.
- without humus, nutrients are washed away and life in the soil declines, the soil turns acid and more organic matter is destroyed.
- the soil no longer holds together, salts build up and erosion increases and quickens at up to 17 times the rate at which it is formed.
- the depleted soils require ever larger inputs of chemicals to produce decreasing levels of yields.
- more fertilizer encourages more weed growth, requiring increased herbicide applications.
- fertilizer encourages fast but weak and sappy growth, making plants vulnerable to insect and fungal attack. Insecticides and fungicides are needed to save the crop.

Intensified animal production has brought widespread diseases that have developed antibiotic resistance

- insecticides indiscriminately wipe out most insects, pests and pollinators, reducing biodiversity both above and below ground.
- herbicides wash into the water supply, giving rise to increased cancer rates and hormonal changes in wildlife and humans that lead to birth defects, gender imbalance and developmental problems.
- plant and animal species become extinct.
- nitrous oxide, a greenhouse gas, is generated from fertilized fields while nitrous acid contributes to acid rain.
- the reduced water retention in soil leads to rapid runoff and flooding after heavy rains.

None of the costs of these side effects of industrial agriculture is charged back to the perpetrators.

Intensified animal production – factory farming – has brought its own problems: widespread diseases that have developed new levels of virulence and antibiotic resistance and skyrocketing rates of food poisoning. Food-borne illness in the US, according to the Center for Disease Control, now kills 9,000 people a year. UK reported cases of food poisoning rose 500% between 1988 and 1998. Animal husbandry, the relationship between the producer and the domestic food animal, has been replaced by levels of animal suffering without historical precedent.

Alongside all this, subsidies to "efficient" modern intensive agriculture have never been higher in Europe or the US. The real cost to the taxpayer of subsidies and cleaning up the mess intensive agriculture causes is estimated to be equal to 40% on the average family's food bill, or about $50 per week.

Pesticide usage creates alarming figures. In 1990, the WHO estimated that there were 3 million acute pesticide poisonings in the developing world, of which 220,000 were fatal. Revised figures indicate 25 million poisoning cases. In the US 20,000 farm workers suffer acute pesticide poisoning every year. Pesticides and herbicides "bioaccumulate," moving up the food chain, often ending up in mothers' milk. The milk of Inuit mothers is so high in residues that it is officially classed as "hazardous waste."

The destruction of habitat by monoculture reduces environmental niches. Extinction is the result, perhaps even of species that have not yet been discovered. Communities themselves suffer extinction in the face of intensification. Rural population declines, communities and the businesses that serve them collapse.

But that's what we have to do to feed ourselves, say many experts. The world, to them, is not too high a price to pay for human survival.

An agricultural monocultural system that can't make money without subsidies, washes

Agricultural intensification is justified based on false costs

away the land, undermines biodiversity and is dependent on fossil fuels for its machinery and chemicals is unsustainable... and inefficient. The sole justification of agricultural intensification has been based on falsified costs.

Small farms produce more food per hectare or acre than large farms; they just do it with more people and lower chemical inputs. A large monoculture farm may produce more corn per acre, but this crude measure doesn't take into account the livestock on a small farm that provide food and manure, bees that pollinate and provide honey and the fewer chemicals used. Many small farms "intercrop," planting a secondary crop between the rows of a main crop, operating with a flexibility not available to monoculture. The 1992 US Agricultural census described the "Inverse Farm Size-Productivity Relationship" and showed that farms under 27

The World Bank now supports smaller-scale farming and ecourages land reform

acres were 10 times more productive in cash output per acre than farms larger than 6,000 acres. Even the World Bank now supports smaller-scale farming and encourages land reform to place small farmers on inefficient large landholdings. True "intensification" of agriculture is when a farmer is in intimate contact with the land, the wildlife and the environment and maximizes only output sustainably.

So why is corporate industrialized farming so powerful?

- Someone else pays the true cost of environmental damage, loss of biodiversity and harm to human health.
- A greater proportion of subsidies goes to the largest farms.
- Many big farms belong to multinationals which can operate at a loss because their real profit comes from trading and processing the farm produce. They also receive tax breaks that small farmers do not.
- Government policy makers are the natural allies of the large oil, chemical, pharmaceutical and agricultural equipment lobbyists. So are "industrial" farmers.

Consumers and taxpayers pay the price for lower quality food and a deteriorating environment. If the true cost of food were transparent, if polluters had to pay for the harm they caused and if soil was seen as an asset that had to be preserved for future generations then industrial agriculture would end.

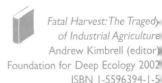

Fatal Harvest: The Tragedy of Industrial Agriculture
Andrew Kimbrell (editor)
Foundation for Deep Ecology 2002
ISBN 1-5596394-1-5

DEADLY DISEASES

the bomb ticks on

In Victorian Britain, the discovery of pathogenic bacteria led to the creation of London's sewer system. Removing people from contact with their own excrement was the most effective way to reduce levels of diseases such as typhoid and cholera. The world agreed and sewage systems around the globe were modeled on London's example.

However, in modern agriculture exposing animals to the excrement of their fellows is commonplace. The intense crowding of cattle feedlots leads to the contamination of beef and milk with *E.coli* O157:H7. Poultry manure is fed to cattle for extra protein – this leads to infection with *Salmonella*. In the US the amounts of manure from farm animals is 10 times that produced by the human population and bypasses the usual sanitation system, making it the single largest cause of river pollution. After hamburgers, waterborne contamination is, inevitably, the next largest cause of *E.coli* infection.

Chicken in cages stacked on wire mesh floors drop excrement onto their neighbors below. "People want cheap chicken," argue the producers. In Sweden, the government announced that if *Salmonella* were found on chicken farms the entire flock would be slaughtered. So, chicken farmers cleaned up their act and *Salmonella* was eliminated. The extra cost of running a clean system was estimated at $8 million per year. The saving to the health system was $28 million. Most *Salmonella* cases in Sweden now occur with returning tourists who picked up the infection abroad. Swedish chicken sells at a premium in other Nordic countries.

In England in late 1988, Health Minister Edwina Currie remarked that "most of the egg production in this country" was contaminated

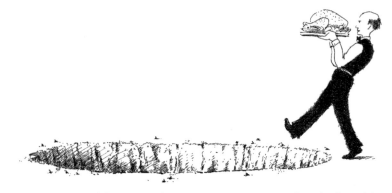

with *Salmonella*, and urged Brits to cook eggs thoroughly. Egg sales fell and she was fired. Two months later, a confidential government report

Up to 2 million *Salmonella* infections a year result from eating eggs and chickens in the UK

was leaked. It stated that up to two million infections a year result from the eating of eggs and chickens in the UK. Between one third and two thirds of all chickens were infected.

A 2002 Consumer Reports test of 484 fresh chickens bought in 25 cities found that half were contaminated with *Campylobacter* or *Salmonella*. 90% of the *Campylobacter* and 34% of the *Salmonella* bacteria had developed antibiotic resistance, increasing the likelihood that infection in humans will not respond to antibiotic treatment. Antibiotics and antimicrobials have made it possible to keep sick animals alive in these grim conditions, allowing pathogens to develop resistance. These mutations have brought suffering and death to consumers around the world.

In June 2001 ConAgra, one of the world's largest agribusiness corporations, recalled 19 million pounds (76 million hamburgers) of *E.coli*-contaminated beef that was produced on intensive feed lots and slaughtered in their highly mechanized slaughterhouses. The *Denver Post* commented: "If 19 million pounds of meat distributed to half of this country had been contaminated with a deadly strain of *E.coli* bacteria by terrorists, we'd go nuts. But when it's done by a *Fortune* 100 corporation, we continue to buy it and feed it to our kids."

There are 61 deaths and 73,000 cases of *E.coli* 0157:H7 poisoning in the US every year. In Britain, where fewer than 60 people have died of the human variant of mad cow disease in the past decade, the entire beef industry was nearly closed down.

"It's time for the Congress to take a good, hard look at food safety policies," said Wenonah Hauter, director of Public Citizen's Critical Mass Energy and Environment Program. "The ConAgra recall is not an aberration. It is another example of a food safety system that is teetering on the brink of collapse."

The Swedes have shown that fecal contamination and the spread of disease are not inevitable in meat production. Better hygiene led to the elimination of typhoid and cholera in Victorian Britain. By not applying the same understanding to our food production we have simply replaced water-borne fecal diseases with new food-borne fecal diseases. The principle of prevention as applied to human sewage has not been applied to meat production and consumers pay the price in disease, disability and death.

• The FAO has stated that cattle fed on pasture have 1/100th the level of *E.coli* 0157:H7 as cattle fed on concentrated food such as corn, soy and ground up animal products. Organic cattle feed on pasture and hay. Organic chickens are not stacked up and exposed to fecal contamination.

It Was Probably Something You Ate:
A Practical Guide to Avoiding and
Surviving Foodborne Illness
Nicols Fox
Penguin 1999
ISBN 0-1402779-9-4

THE (NOT-SO?) GREEN REVOLUTION

when "green" isn't good

Norman Borlaug, the "Father of the Green Revolution," which was brought to the developing world back in the 1970s, has called for a "Second Green Revolution." But do we need another one? What was the first and how successful was it?

Back in the '60s, amidst dire warnings of global famines, Norman Borlaug developed his "miracle

Between 1970 and 1990 the number of hungry people went up

wheat" that was set to change grain yields in some of the world's most vulnerable countries.

The "Green Revolution" depended on short-stalk wheat and rice. Grain crops naturally grow on stalks that are several feet high,

supported by strong root structures. The high plant shades out competition from weeds and also provides straw for animal bedding, thatching and other uses. New hybrid varieties developed had very short stalks and limited root networks, thus allowing the plant to concentrate its energy on seed production. As long as plenty of chemical weed killers and fertilizers were applied bigger crops could be harvested. Irrigation was necessary as these crops couldn't survive dry conditions.

This new crop came to India and, indeed, where food shortages had once been forecast, yields of cereal grains went up and India began to export wheat. But the news had a sting in its tail. Between 1970 and 1990 (the two decades of major Green Revolution advances) the number of hungry people in the world actually went up from 536 million to 597 million. The mere existence of food has never been a guarantee that everyone eats. If it were then there would be no hunger in the United States (33.6 million Americans are food insecure, hungry or at risk of hunger) or India, both food exporting-countries. Poverty is the main cause of hunger; loss of land to grow one's own food on is the other.

The practicalities of the Green Revolution were hard for smaller farmers. They couldn't afford the new seeds and chemicals so were forced off their land while larger farmers prospered. Chemicals replaced labor; small farmers and farm laborers joined the ranks of the unemployed and hungry. The fertility and humus content of the soil fell. This decline in fertility meant farmers in India had to use more and more fertilizer each year just to maintain the same yields. Profit margins were squeezed as higher yields brought falling prices against a background of higher fertilizer cost.

As the fertility and mineral content of the soil have fallen, so have the levels of iron, zinc and Vitamin A in the food produced. Anemia and other deficiency diseases abound. These losses counteract any gains in carbohydrate availability. Consumption of fruits, vegetables and legumes has also fallen. In Bangladesh before the Green Revolution, there were over 100 types of green plants that flourished alongside rice in the paddies providing dietary

33.6 million Americans are food insecure, hungry or at risk of hunger

beta-carotenes, iron and folic acid. The use of herbicides has killed these plants. Rice production increased, but extra blindness, anemia and birth defects resulted from the loss of these supplementary foods. Six million children die each year of malnutrition. India and Bangladesh share a high proportion of that figure.

Was the Green Revolution worth it? In 1993 a study of farms in South India found that the productivity and profitability of "ecological farms" was equal to that of chemical-intensive farms that followed the Green Revolution. Profits, however, were shared among a larger number of people on "ecological farms." Soil erosion and depletion of fertility were all

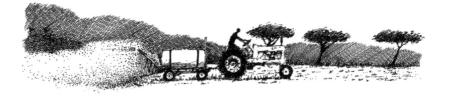

higher on the intensive farms. Indian farmers who cannot repay debt incurred to purchase chemical inputs and hybrid seeds commit suicide in the thousands each year – in July 2004 the Prime Minister announced a $1,136 payment to the families of such farmers – small compensation for the loss of a breadwinner.

The Green Revolution has gone flat. Norman Borlaug hopes that a "Second Green Revolution" will be based on genetic

> We can't solve problems by using the same kind of thinking we used when we created them

engineering – that modified crops will one day deliver higher yields with lower fertilizer and pesticide inputs. Engineering crops to grow in

saline soil is part of this dream. But saline soil is caused by use of nitrates and over-irrigation, two essentials of the Green Revolution. His call is enthusiastically supported by chemical companies such as Monsanto, Novartis and Dupont, as well as the World Bank and other international agencies. They claim hunger and starvation can only be beaten with the tools of biotechnology. Albert Einstein wrote: "We can't solve problems by using the same kind of thinking we used when we created them."

So far all progress has been theoretical, with the word "might" used alongside all the anticipated miracles of genetic engineering since the 1980s. For the 5,000 children a day who die of malnutrition in India, that is small comfort.

SRI (System of Rice Intensification) rice production is a new intensive and organic method that is generating yields double those of Green Revolution techniques. It works by planting rice plants further apart and irrigating little if at all. Yields increase by double or even more – labor costs are higher but no fertilizers or herbicides costs are incurred and seed costs are halved. SRI has been debunked and attacked by advocates of genetic engineered rice, but it has spread from Madagascar, where it originated, to most rice-growing nations – in China tripling of yields has been achieved.

• The regions of Andhra Pradesh and Punjab, India's two leading agricultural regions, suffer high rates of agricultural suicide as farmers struggle to meet crippling interest rates on grain and chemical purchases.

• Irrigated and chemically fertilized land suffers salination and has to be taken out of production. 6% of India's agricultural land is now useless and the rate of loss is increasing.

• A farmer using pesticides and fertilizers uses 12 calories of energy from fossil fuels to produce one calorie of food energy. A subsistence farmer with a hoe uses one calorie of energy to produce 20 calories of food. A sustainable "revolution" lies somewhere between these extremes of high and low-tech farming.

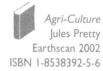

Agri-Culture
Jules Pretty
Earthscan 2002
ISBN 1-8538392-5-6

FOOD MILES AND THE FOOD CHAIN

going far?

In the 19th century, when oranges were only available for a few months of the year, wealthy country-house owners built large greenhouses, or orangeries, to extend the season for these luxury goods. Now, thanks to cheap fuel, yesterday's luxuries are today's "commodities" and oranges and orange juice are available all the year round. But have we gone too far?

New Jersey license plates proudly proclaim "The Garden State" remembering a time when

> The 1997 Census of Agriculture showed that nearly every state has seen a decline in vegetable farms

the metropolises of New York and Philadelphia obtained most of their vegetables from their horticultural neighbor. Not any more. The 1997 Census of Agriculture showed that every state except California has seen a decline in the number of vegetable farms, with Texas and Florida showing the largest falls. Are Americans eating fewer vegetables? No. They're just bringing them in from Mexico, Honduras, Salvador, Chile and further abroad. In 1995 the US imported $10 billion worth of horticultural products such as fruit and vegetables each year. By 2003 that figure had more than doubled to $21 billion.

Fossil fuels are the foundation of our modern food supply. Cheap oil is an essential ingredient in the manufacture and transport of chemical fertilizers, pesticides and as fuel for agricultural machinery. Once food has left the farm, high levels of fuel are used to transport it long distances before it reaches the consumer. This system is, oddly, promoted as "efficient" and it assumes that fossil fuel supplies are infinite and that oil prices will remain stable. The true cost of transporting food over great distances, however, is not that low, particularly if we consider the massive future costs of global warming, caused by CO_2 emissions and oil shortages.

Transport by road and by air uses up lots of fuel – the "cheapness" of which is artificial. Roads are built by governments using taxpayers' money and then provided "free" for transport use. The weight of heavy trucks wears out roads, increasing the frequency and cost of repairs. Aviation fuel is untaxed, giving airfreight a strong competitive advantage. An airline pays $1 per gallon for fuel, while a trucking company must pay $1.75. Airfreight burns 50 gallons of fuel to carry the amount of food for which a ship would burn one gallon, or highway transport six gallons. Without such "subsidized" air transport and free highways, a very different pattern of food growing and distribution would emerge.

More than one-third of all truck traffic is carrying food. By the time the food reaches the supermarkets, its production and distribution has produced eight tons of carbon dioxide emissions per household.

So what's the solution?

The WTO opposes any "restraint" on free global trade. Any tariff barriers against imported food would be struck down as unfair and anti-competitive. But there are other ways to reduce food miles.

There is already a growing trend toward localized food systems with farmers' markets, home delivery services and community

There is a growing trend toward localized food systems

supported agriculture. The more customers appreciate the benefits of fresh, locally produced food, the more supermarkets will have to find ways to fulfill that demand. Where they have tried, they encounter a conflict between their structure – designed for centralized economies of scale – and the need for more sensitive locally devolved buying power. Seasonal foods are also better appreciated now. Anyone who has tasted fresh homegrown asparagus knows that no price discount can make the imported alternative taste better. The term "imported" could finally be losing its cachet.

Environmental taxes on aviation fuel and road use would help tip the balance in favor of local and regional produce. However, taxes that threaten people's love affair with air travel and cars are political vote-losers. Subsidizing local production and supporting targets for increasing domestic production would, perhaps, prove less politically sensitive. Surely, growing low-value subsidized soybeans, corn and cotton

> Environmental taxes on aviation fuel and road use would help tip the balance for regional produce

for export and then importing high-value produce such as fresh fruit and vegetables is economic nonsense.

• In the 1970s, UK fruit producers were subsidized to grub out apple trees. Half of Britain's apple orchards disappeared. Imports from Chile, South Africa, the USA, New Zealand and Europe, often coated in preservative fungicides such as Captan or diphenylamine, filled the gap. The consequent loss to the British rural economy hinged on a few pennies per pound saving on cheaper imports. In 2002 local fruit production begun making a (government-subsidized) comeback. Consumer taste has moved on from the days when Golden Delicious was the popular ideal.

The Food Miles Report: The dangers of long-distance food transport
Angela Paxton
SAFE Alliance 1994
ISBN 1-8997790-5-1

SUPERMARKETS

one-stop shopping?

The self-service store is a modern creation, made possible through the advances in food processing, packaging and distribution of the 1950s. No longer tied to the ham slicer, the cheese wire and the cracker barrel, grocers could concentrate on stocking the shelves and taking the money. Chains such as A&P and Safeway also accrued considerable negotiating power. They negotiated lower prices from suppliers and so shifted the balance of power from the producer to the retailer. The consumer – the retailer's primary route to profit – liked it. The pressure on suppliers for cheapness led to corner-cutting, particularly in meat production, where what the buyer didn't see they didn't know – until *Salmonella*, *E.coli* and BSE appeared and the hidden cost of bargain prices had to be paid.

By the 1970s, a handful of supermarkets controlled most food sales. It was said that 15 men decided what the rest of the population ate. It wasn't quite that simple – but those 15 men did have immense power and dictated what appeared on the shelves: the brand leader, the number two and the supermarket's own-label version. Any brand that didn't make the grade either disappeared or reinvented itself as a "gourmet" brand to carve out a niche in specialty food shops. Small independent grocers went out of business in droves. Food manufacturers merged into giant conglomerates,

It was said 15 men decided what the rest of the population ate

trying to match the increased power of the big stores. As supermarkets expanded to provide hardware, clothing, housewares, drugstore products, newspapers and magazines, their impact adversely affected main street retailers in all sectors. The "Wal-Mart effect" of decaying business districts in towns across the country was part of the price, along with reduced food quality and debased animal and employee welfare standards. The desire for year-round availability led to rising food imports, which often replaced domestic production, with costs to the domestic economy as well as increased fossil fuel usage. With 9% of every retail dollar spent, Wal-Mart dominates the US retail scene and is a force worldwide (though Britain's Tesco takes 12%). With 1.1 million employees, it is the largest US private employer, it is China's biggest customer, buying $12 billion per year, and is introducing RFID (radio frequency identification

Research shows that consumers only remember what a few of the most popular food items cost

tags) to its products to improve stock control, save $8 billion on warehouse labor and, most importantly, when combined with loyalty card data, to walk and talk customers through the store, alerting them to special offers on products for which they have a known preference, helping them to optimize their purchasing as it guides

them to the checkout. But, with resistance to Wal-Mart store openings in California and a lawsuit in Mexico for monopolistic practices, the path to global domination faces challenges.

The supermarkets' influence is also a psychological one. Walk in and the first thing you see is fresh produce. This sets the consumer's impression of the whole store. It's also the perishable food that brings the customer back to the store. After fresh produce the other perishable foods that shoppers regularly buy are bread and milk. These are usually found at the opposite end of the store, requiring shoppers to cross the entire store. "Impulse purchases" are encouraged by placing selected items at the end of aisles. Deep price discounts on "Known Value Items" such as milk, sliced bread, cornflakes and canned tomatoes cash in on research showing that consumers only remember what a few of the most popular food items actually cost. By making sure these always look cheap, supermarkets create the overall impression of low prices without giving too much away.

Organic and high quality food
By the 1990s supermarkets had developed "loyalty cards," which provided details on

consumer preferences. One of their discoveries was that consumers who bought just one organic item were likely to spend twice as much as other shoppers per store visit. These are the consumers that supermarkets want – those who appreciate quality and don't buy solely on price. No sooner had they identified these customers, than the supermarkets noticed they were visiting their stores less often. Organic home delivery of seasonal vegetables and farmers' markets were blamed. Organic retail chains grew rapidly. In Britain, the supermarkets sought out organic suppliers and introduced organic ranges, many under their own label. In the US, they relied much more on suppliers who would merchandise a natural foods section – a "store within a store." A niche existed which was quickly filled by regional natural foods supermarket chains such as Mrs. Gooch's in So. California, Bread and Circus in New England, Freshfields in the mid- Atlantic states, Whole Foods Market in Texas and Wild Oats across the western states. During the 1990s, Whole Foods Market, with Wall Street backing, acquired all these other chains except Wild Oats and conquered the demographic high ground right across the country. Unlike in Britain, where the supermarkets could skim the cream of the organic retail market, in the US two dedicated organic chains made market penetration more difficult. As organic and high quality become more synonymous, the high-end consumers as well as the middle-income, committed consumers migrate away from the mainstream supermarkets towards the offerings of the organic supers.

The balance of power has shifted: no longer do 15 male supermarket buyers decide what we eat. Every purchase at the checkout is a vote recorded for a particular product, and if supermarkets ignore their customers they will shop elsewhere. A useful side effect is that the corruptibility of supermarket buyers is checked by the fact that consumer preferences are fully understood and are the main driver for what items are stocked.

• Since the 1950s, the proportion of income Americans spend on food has dropped from 25% to 8%, while real incomes have gone up. Even if everyone switched to organic food, that proportion wouldn't exceed 10%. All the data suggests that supermarkets must provide the customer with organic, high-quality, locally sourced food if they are to regain a larger share of people's spending.

TASTES FAMILIAR

fooling your taste buds

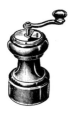

We all learned in school that there are four tastes: sweet, salty, sour and bitter. There's another taste, however, that is the favorite of food technologists and mass caterers. It's called *umami*, and translates as "meaty" or "savory" and is conveyed by several naturally occurring substances, including glutamate – an amino acid present in protein-rich foods.

The FDA estimates that 2% of the US population is MSG reactive; other claim up to 50%

Umami was always a part of Japanese cuisine, with *dashi kombu* or seaweed broth, used as the base for miso soup, noodle broth and other staples. In Europe, *umami* is tasted in chicken stock, beef extract and aged cheeses such as cheddar. Tomatoes, mushrooms, baby peas or freshly picked sweet corn all have small quantities of glutamic acid that turns into more complex, but less flavorsome, proteins as the vegetable ripens. That's why we pick them young, while the flavor is at its peak – a signal that nutritious proteins are present.

Back in the 1920s Japanese scientist Kikunae Ikeda studied kombu seaweed and isolated the glutamic acid molecule that was the essence of umami flavor. He developed a cheap way to get glutamic acid, crystallizing it and manufacturing its salt, monosodium glutamate (MSG). Ikeda then founded the Ajinomoto Corporation, the world's leading manufacturer of artificial flavorings and sweeteners. Vast quantities of MSG are now made using acid hydrolysis. A protein source, (usually defatted soybean meal), is boiled in hydrochloric acid. The acid breaks down the proteins, some of which form glutamic acid.

MSG use spread worldwide. From being an unacknowledged element in people's diet, MSG attained unprecedented levels of consumption. No research into MSG's safety was done before adding it to the food supply – people didn't bother with such things back then.

But by the 1970s the "Chinese Restaurant Syndrome" had emerged – numbness, palpitations, headaches and abdominal pains after eating large quantities of MSG. People with allergies or asthma were found to react adversely to small quantities of MSG because glutamic acid also acts as a neurotransmitter in the brain. In babies, as well as unborn babies, glutamic acid passes the brain blood barrier, causing damage to the brain and nervous system. It is now banned in baby foods. It could also pass the barrier in people with hypertension, low blood sugar, diabetes, Alzheimer's, infections and strokes.

• The FDA estimates that 2% of the US population is MSG reactive; others put sensitivity to MSG as high as 15% to 20% – that's about 50,000,000 people; Dr. George Schwartz, author of In Bad Taste: The MSG Symptom Complex, believes the numbers are much higher, perhaps 40% to 50%.

Even a healthy person, having consumed three grams of MSG on an empty stomach, could develop MSG-related symptoms. A

Even a healthy person can show symtoms with 3 grams of MSG

serving of a typical meal with food containing glutamate has only half a gram of MSG, so a healthy person would have to eat six servings before feeling effects. Some snack foods, however, such as dry-roasted nuts, flavored potato chips and certain puffed snacks, have much higher levels of MSG. So in one quick snack the high doses of MSG trigger a rapid increase in blood glutamate levels and adverse affects are likely to be experienced more quickly and intensely.

If MSG were invented today it would probably not gain approval for use in food. It is, however, now universal. The MSG industry has set up the Glutamate Association to fund research into defending the safety of their product at a time when negative opinion threatens to lead to it being banned, or, at least, to being clearly labelled on food products and restaurant menus.

Instead MSG is hidden under many names: "Hydrolyzed vegetable protein," "plant protein extract," "natural flavoring," "seasoning," "spices" or "vegetable bouillon."

The use of MSG has enabled producers to create cheap, flavorless food

Good food tastes good without the need for chemical aids. The use of MSG in its various guises has enabled processors and producers to create cheap, flavorless food and cover up its deficiencies with MSG and artificial flavorings. Worse, because of the palate's instinctive attraction to glutamic acid, the use of MSG seduces our tastes away from wholesome food to less natural alternatives.

• In the late '60s, some Chinese restaurants would put a pot of MSG on tables for diners to sprinkle on their food.

• Organic food regulations prohibit the use of MSG, hydrolyzed protein or any ingredient which contains MSG.

In Bad Taste: The MSG Symptom Complex
George R. Schwartz
Health Press (NM) 1999
ISBN: 0-929173-30-9

Excitotoxins: The Taste That Kills
Russell L. Blaylock, M.D.
Health Press (NM), 1994
ISBN 0-929173-25-2

PERSUASION – ADS

banning truth about healthy eating

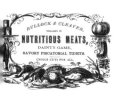

Why do we eat so much junk food? Is it fair to blame the advertisers just because we can't control our decadent appetites for sugary, fattening food? Are kids being brainwashed by advertising or is their laziness and obesity really the fault of parents who drive them everywhere, use the television or game player as a cheap babysitter and give them fast food because they're too busy to cook them a proper meal?

What do we really know about the food we eat? The National Advertising Review Council (NARC) was set up in 1971 to protect consumers from misleading or factually inaccurate advertising. It is made up of people from the media, the advertising industry and the advertisers themselves and its mission statement is that the advertising industry should be self-regulating, increase public trust in advertising, regulate disputes between advertisers and keep the government out of regulating advertising. In 1957 Vance Packard's book *The Hidden Persuaders*, shocked Americans with its exposé of how subtle psychological techniques were used to sell cake mixes, cars and soap. This was in the relatively crude days of "subliminal advertising" (where the words like "drink cola" would be flashed

Why do we eat so much junk food? Is it fair to blame the ads?

across the screen for a fraction of a second) and rather simple motivational and aspirational hooks. Vance Packard believed that if people could understand the techniques they could resist them, and public confidence in advertisers plummeted in the 1960s. The NARC was set up to restore trust.

But most kids haven't read *The Hidden Persuaders,* and the techniques have become much more sophisticated as psychological understanding of what motivates us has increased. "Spin" in politics and business is commonplace and an essential ingredient in successful competition, whether for votes or dollars at the checkout. With TV ads that merge seamlessly with the characters in the cartoon shows that kids are watching, it is no surprise that one-third of American kids are brand-aware by the age of three.

Criticism of the advertising industry has hit home though, and there has been a positive reaction.

Most people will have difficulty squaring ad guidelines with what their kids actually see on TV

Son of NARC, or CARU (Children's Advertising Review Unit) was set up in 1974 to "ensure the truth and accuracy of child-directed advertising."

Not everyone was happy that this self-regulatory body was effective in controlling the abuse and manipulation of young minds. Even NARC had to admit that the huge increase in obesity among children in the 1980s and 1990s indicated that advertisers of fattening products had failed to stem the tide of blubber.

On May 28, 2004 NARC published a white paper of *Guidance for Food Advertising Self-Regulation.* It calls for greater understanding of advertising self-regulation and points out that the food industry has put nutritional information on menus and removed transfats from marketed snacks.

The guidelines are clear and contain key recommendations that most people will have difficulty in squaring with what they, or their kids actually see on TV. Here are a few key rules:
- Advertising... should not mislead children about benefits (such as) the acquisition of strength, status, popularity, growth, proficiency and intelligence.
- Representation of food products should... encourage... healthy development of the child and development of good nutritional practices.

- Advertisements representing mealtime should clearly depict the role of the product within the framework of a balanced diet.
- Program personalities, live or animated, should not be used to sell products in or adjacent to programs primarily directed to children in which the same personality or characters appear.

Watch kids' TV for an hour or so and compare the ideals to the reality. CARU has been successful in keeping regulation of advertising in advertisers' hands. Reading their white paper summaries of cited cases show how often the guidelines are violated and how, by the time CARU does anything about it, the ad campaign is over. Typical is the case of an ad where a kid says "I only know one kid who eats wheat bread" – a visual appears of a little girl wearing glasses – the boy says, "What a little dork." The offending advertiser promised to take CARU's guidelines into consideration in future ads. The essential toothlessness of all self-regulatory advertising, whether aimed at adults or kids, lies in the fact that the regulatory activity occurs after the advertising damage has been done. There is no punishment, just a gentle slap on the wrist. An advertiser who is challenged can go through a prolonged appeal process by simply submitting a check for $500 payable to the Better Business Bureau. In the context of the millions that are spent on advertising campaigns, a few hundred dollars is a small price to pay to defer the final arrival of a mild rebuke.

Unsurprising then that, by the 1990s, challenges by consumer advocacy groups had pretty much dried up (why bother when no effective preventive action is taken?) and most cases now are between competitors complaining about the "my product is better than yours" type of ad.

Advertising faces bigger problems. As adults and kids take control, in the digital age, of their viewing and information choices, advertisers will find it less easy to reach them or persuade them using time-tested psychological techniques.

It is doubtful if self-regulation or governmental regulation can be any more effective in the future than it has been in the past in helping kids or adults to understand the real issues about nutrition and health and avoid obesity. Advertisers would be wasting their money if they exhorted their customers to "Eat less fat" or "Cut down on Big Macs" or "Drink less Coke." Why pay for advertising unless your message is to encourage consumers to divert more of their expenditure in the direction of your product? The highest profit margins, and therefore the highest advertising budgets, are for fast food, soft drinks and snacks.

• The world's biggest advertiser, sometimes criticized for associating soft drink consumption with glamour, upward social mobility and success, is Coca-Cola. Neville Isdell, the Irish-born Chairman and CEO, newly appointed in June 2004, took the bull by the horns. After saying, "scapegoating certain foods which are good or bad" wouldn't solve the obesity

> The highest profit margins, and the highest ad budgets, are for fast food, soft drinks and snacks

crisis; he identified what might be called "The Coke Paradox."

"Coca-Cola's vested interest is in a healthy population: Healthier consumers are going to be good for us. They will grow older, healthier, wealthier and hopefully therefore able to buy more from us. Which at the end of the day, let's face it, is our goal." So, drink more Dasani perhaps?

Coercion: Why We Listen to What They Say
Douglas Rushkoff
Riverhead Books 2000
ISBN 1-5732282-9-X

SWEET NOTHINGS

the truth about sugar

The average American eats 145 pounds of sugar every year – that's about 28 teaspoons a day. At the beginning of the 20th century sugar was still a rare luxury, with average consumption levels at around five pounds per year, less than one teaspoon per day. This spectacular 2,800% rise in sugar consumption is one of the most significant changes in our modern diet.

Sugar from sugar cane is one of our oldest foods, originating in India 5,000 years ago. Before its introduction to the West by Crusaders, honey and fruit were our occasional and seasonal sources of simple sugars such as sucrose, glucose and fructose. It was Christopher Columbus who carried a sugar cane plant to the Caribbean, and slave labor ensured that it remained cheap.

Sugar is sucrose, a combination of one glucose and one fructose molecule. Glucose is the only sugar that our body can use directly. Fructose is converted into glycogen and stored for later use in the liver. When the liver detects a drop in blood sugar level, it converts glycogen into glucose.

How is sugar converted to fat?

We should have about 80 calories of glucose (three teaspoons) in our blood and another 300 calories stored as glycogen. We need at least 600 calories a day just to keep going. The backup supply comes from body fat, where a further 100,000 calories are on standby, ready to be converted quickly into glucose. This interchangeability – converting sugars into fats and vice versa – gives us great flexibility and means we can survive on a wide range of foods.

How does sugar make you fat?

When we have a sudden intake of sugar, say a canned soft drink that contains 100 calories or four teaspoons of sugars, two or three teaspoons of glucose go straight into the bloodstream, doubling the blood sugar level. The pancreas releases insulin into the blood to mop up excess sugars, some of which are converted to fats and put into storage. If more sugar is eaten, the fat has little chance to get converted back into sugar and so accumulates. Obesity is a sign that there is more than the 100,000 calories worth of fat that a healthy person needs in reserve.

Insulin Resistance Syndrome and Diabetes

Continued and sudden intakes of sugar lead to frequent insulin releases into the bloodstream. This leads to "insulin resistance syndrome," where it takes more and more insulin to get

Sugar is the main cause of dental decay and gum disease

the blood sugar level back down to normal. The pancreas continues to produce insulin and too much blood sugar is mopped up, resulting in "hypoglycemia," or low blood sugar, the symptoms of which are stress, tiredness, anxiety and cravings for sweets. The pancreas produces as much insulin as it can, but eventually stops

producing insulin at all. Type II diabetes is the result. When diabetes accompanies high blood pressure and obesity, heart disease usually follows. High sugar consumption, inactivity, stress and smoking all increase the risk of obesity, heart attack and stroke.

And then there's our teeth. Sugar is the main cause of dental decay and gum disease. Toothbrushing can help, as can fluoride, but by far the most effective way to prevent decay is to avoid sugar, or to consume it rarely and only with meals. It has also been shown that cancer cells thrive on glucose. Some therapies work by starving the cancerous cells of sugar.

So, it's the "surges" in blood glucose level that cause most of the trouble, rather than the sugar itself. Indeed, one of the key functions of blood is to carry sugar, in the form of glucose, around the body. The brain uses more than 300 calories a day, up to half of the glucose in the bloodstream. When the blood sugar level is low, the brain cells, muscles and nerves of the body cannot function correctly and fatigue irritability, nervousness and faintness result. In extreme forms it exists as bad temper, neurotic behavior and paranoia.

Sugar displaces more nutritious foods

Sugar satisfies a need for calories but eating more wholesome foods would mean vitamins, minerals, fiber, antioxidants and other micronutrients would also be gained – all of which encourage good health and a strong immune function. Artificial sweeteners such as aspartame, cyclamates and saccharin are equally undesirable (see chapter "Obesity"). They may replace the calories of sugar, but they can also cause health problems. There is an alternative. The leaves of Stevia rebaudiana, a Brazilian plant, produce stevioside, a non-calorific natural sweetener, but lobbying by the manufacturers of other sweeteners has blocked its approval.

Thus, keeping blood sugar levels even is the key to preventing cardiovascular disease, diabetes, obesity, tooth decay and cancer. But sugar is so genuinely addictive that many people struggle with their craving for it.

The safest way to eat sugar is in small quantities with foods that will delay its rapid assimilation and so reduce the extreme swings in blood sugar, energy level and mood: high-fiber foods, for example, such as wholegrain bread, legumes, vegetables and whole cereal products. Apple crumble will have a far milder impact than a glass of apple juice with the same level of sugars.

Without glucose and oxygen, our food and breath, we would die in minutes. Sugar certainly makes many foods taste better. But too much of this particular good thing can wreak havoc.

• In 1942, when annual production of fizzy soft drinks was about 60 12-ounce servings per person, the American Medical Association's Council on Foods and Nutrition stated: "The Council believes it would be in the interest of the public health for all practical means to be taken to limit consumption of sugar in any form in which it fails to be combined with significant proportions of other foods of high nutritive quality."

• Today, Americans consume on average ten times the 1942 level of soft drinks and the rest of the world is fast catching up.

The Schwarzbein Principle: The Truth About Weight Loss, Health and Aging
Diana Schwarzbein, Nancy Devile
Health Communications 1999
ISBN 1-5587468-0-3

COMMODITY MARKETS

reality distorted

The dollar turnover of the largest corporations exceeds that of many of the world's countries. So, a democracy, such as Chile, can be dominated easily by commercial interests. These, inevitably, place the interests of Chile's voters low in their list of priorities.

It is, perhaps, even more alarming that America's largest corporations are far richer and more powerful than US government departments such as the US Department

> Eisenhower warned against yielding to public pressure for wasteful public funding of agriculture

of Agriculture, the Environment Protection Agency and the Food and Drug Administration. With power divided among 50 states, individual senators and representatives, particularly those who chair important committees, can have inordinate power. The voter, even the political party, is often sidelined in this process.

In 1950, 25% of US tax income came from corporations. That figure is now 10%. "Corporate Welfare," giving public money to corporations, was not even discussed in 1950. In 1960, when President Eisenhower handed over power to John Kennedy, he warned against yielding to pressure for wasteful public funding of agriculture and applied research. (In other words, against a system of unsustainable subsidies.) He warned that, "In the councils of government, we must guard against the acquisition of unwarranted influence by the military-industrial complex. The potential for the disastrous rise of misplaced power exists and will persist."

What is "misplaced power?" It is not power that derives from the open market; it has een granted, instead, by government to big business. It excludes smaller companies, which must watch helplessly as their big competitors are helped to become even bigger. The level of consolidation in military and food industries now rivals that of Communist Russia.

Billions of dollars annually are fed to Cargill, which controls most of America's grain and soybean trade. Its main "competitor," ADM (Archer Daniels Midland), receives billions in subsidies to convert unwanted subsidized corn into ethanol to be burned with gasoline (see chapter "Energy").

But the support of Congress-picked "winners" doesn't stop at the US border. Billions of dollars a year go into the Market Promotion Program and Export Enhancement Programs to help Cargill and ADM compete against producers elsewhere in the world for contracts for wheat, corn and soybeans. Because Cargill and ADM benefit from subsidized prices, they get the contracts and local producers lose out. The mighty McDonald's corporation and other burger companies expand their global empires on the back of sales of 99¢ hamburgers that would cost three times as much in the absence

of corporate welfare. The entire world market for food has become grossly distorted. Small farmers worldwide go out of business as larger but less efficient producers in rich countries thrive on government handouts.

Economist Stephen Moore of the Cato Institute warns, "Every major US Cabinet department has become a conduit for government funding of

Taxpayers annually pay up to $167 billion to support top corporations

private industry." They conservatively estimate that taxpayers pay about $75 billion per year to support America's largest corporations. Ralph Nader estimates the total value as closer to $167 billion.

In a free society, the market selects ideas for investment. There is freedom from restriction, from coercion and from the use of force. When it is subverted, we don't just lose freedom of choice, we lose our personal freedom. "Creative destruction" is the healthy mechanism whereby businesses with good ideas or products can challenge and replace existing industries. It may create losers, but it also creates winners who are keeping up with changes. If government takes one company's side against its smaller, newer competitors, then society as a whole is the loser.

America is not alone; the establishment of the EU with power vested in the European Commission means that corporate influence can be concentrated in one place, Brussels, rather than in national capitals all over the continent.

Two centuries of sugar subsidies show how easy it is to start out on the path to "corporate welfare" and how fiendishly difficult it is to

In eight EU countries, just one national company controls the entire beet sugar quota

get off. In the Napoleonic Wars the British blockaded France's sugar supplies from Haiti and Louisiana in the hope that a sugar-starved French populace would rise up and overthrow Napoleon. But Napoleon, undaunted, set aside 80,000 acres for sugar beet growing. After Waterloo and the lifting of the blockade,

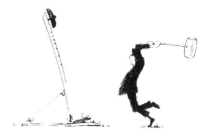

cheaper sugar imports from the West Indies resumed, but the beet sugar industry, farmers and refinery operators, bribed, rioted and eventually forced a settlement that guaranteed them half of France's sugar market, at a permanent cost to the French taxpayer.

With expansion of the Common Market, this policy now pervades the EU. In each of eight countries, just one national company controls the entire national beet sugar quota: in Britain it is British Sugar; in France it is Générai Sucrière. The price of sugar in Europe is three times the world price, protected by tariffs and subsidies worth $2 billion annually. Worse, export subsidies mean that Europe's surplus goes to developing countries, displacing low-cost sugar producers such as Mozambique. So unsubsidized small producers suffer as their export markets are swallowed up by EU sugar. If trade is not fair and open, then everyone loses out – especially the poor.

In the USA things are no better. Every attempt by Congress to eliminate federal sugar price support is defeated by Senators or representatives who have received campaign contributions from the sugar producers. Sugar producers get 30 times more subsidy per acre than wheat producers. The cost to American consumers is $2 billion a year.

In Florida, the main sugar-producing state, alligators suffer endocrine disruption from pesticides used on sugar, leading, alarmingly, to inadequate penis development or even to sex change. 500,000 acres of the Everglades have been drained for sugar production that is blatantly uneconomic.

Taxpayers lose, Third World producers bound by WTO free trade agreements lose, confectionery industry workers in the US lose, too, as confectionery manufacturers move to Canada or Mexico, where sugar sells at the world price. One small but powerful interest group harms fellow citizens, foreign producers and the environment in the scramble for government money.

• Europe's sugar regime "preserves the interests of all the parties concerned. It was deliberately designed to this effect. It must be maintained." The European Sugar Manufacturers' Association.

• "Europe's policies... are putting us at a disadvantage. They are rich and could give us a chance to live." Sugar cane harvester, Mozambique.

The Great EU Sugar Scam
Oxfam Briefing Paper 27
www.oxfam.org.uk/what_we_do/
issues/trade/bp27_sugar.htm

www.oxfam.org

www.nader.org

FAIR TRADE

how much fairer?

We have been taught that free trade is a good thing. However, it is often deeply unfair, or, to use tougher language – unjust and exploitative.

Take chocolate as an example. It is a "premium" food, associated with indulgence and luxury. However, it comes at a price that includes slavery, environmental degradation and poverty.

Imagine the cost of cocoa bean production as $900 per ton. A small farmer who produces 10 tons per year and sells at $1,000 per ton makes a profit of $100 per ton or a total of $1,000. If the cocoa price were $1,100 then he would make $2,000 for his year's work. So, a small 10%

Chocolate comes at a price that includes slavery, environmental degredation and poverty

increase in the cocoa price doubles the farmer's profit. Yet traders insist on keeping prices as low as possible. It is this crucial difference that the international Fairtrade Labeling Organization (FLO) seeks to address by setting "fair" prices.

In 1982, Felix Houphouet-Boigny, the President of the Ivory Coast, the world's largest producer of cocoa beans, boldly announced that cocoa prices were too low and they would not be selling that year's crop. The world markets went crazy and prices soared to $3,000. Satisfied, the Ivory Coast began to sell again and the price settled down. In the next few years USAID, Britain's Overseas Development Agency and their German, Dutch and Swiss counterparts all embarked on a global aid exercise to help small farmers in Honduras, Belize, Papua New Guinea, Solomon Islands, Malaysia and other non-African countries to "reduce poverty" by planting cacao trees. By the early 1990s there was, therefore, global overcapacity in cacao and the price had settled down to less than $1,000. Now, whenever the price starts to rise, the huge spare capacity that has been created kicks into action and the price sags to a level that allows cocoa growers to survive – and little more. The world's leading American, British, German, Dutch and Swiss chocolate manufacturers can sleep easy. There will be no more shocks from Africans with ideas above their station.

Should world prices be allowed to rise and farmers earn a decent profit, the impact on the price of chocolate bars would be minuscule. A $500 per ton increase in cocoa prices on the cost of a large 3 1/2 oz bar of milk chocolate is exactly one cent. Yet an extra $500 per ton to a small producer could make a huge difference to a whole country's health system, education and future investment. So why not allow prices for cocoa to rise? If all a producer country's exports were based on principles of "fair trade," the extra foreign exchange would help reduce their crippling interest burdens and support investment in economic development.

The ruthless logic of commodity markets, supported by unhelpful aid programs, led to the development of a fair trade movement in the early 1990s. FLO was established to ensure that national standards of fair trade were observed in all 17 participating countries. In Britain the Fairtrade Foundation was set up by Oxfam, Christian Aid and other charities to certify fairly traded products to FLO standards. The first product they licensed, in 1994, was Green & Black's Maya Gold

The ruthless logic of commodity markets led to a fair trade push

chocolate, made with cocoa beans grown by the indigenous Maya of Belize. With a five-year rolling contract, cash in advance, a guaranteed fair price and support in obtaining organic certification, the project became a model scheme. Ten years later secondary education in the region has risen from 10% to 90%, herbicide pollution of the rivers is no more, forest cover is increasing along with migratory bird populations, women's status and the status of the Maya in Belize have both been transformed, nutrition has improved and in 2004 alone 500,000 new cacao trees were planted, with full forest shade cover, to satisfy the growth in demand for Maya Gold chocolate. All for a penny or so on the cost of a bar of chocolate.

Fair trade's main focus is on pricing and social conditions:

Pricing – the price of production is set by experts, then a fair trade premium is added to ensure producers get a reasonable return. Payment is in advance, so producers get cash on delivery of goods. Long-term contracts offer security and sustainability to producer cooperatives.

Social – small producer cooperatives must be democratic. Plantation workers must have the

> With even Starbucks selling fair trade coffee, the tentacles of ethical trading are reaching deeper

right to form unions and have decent wages, and health and safety standards. Child labor is prohibited and there must be appropriate programs for environmental sustainability. The most dangerous agrichemicals are not allowed but in practice most fair trade producers are also organic.

Products that comply with Fairtrade Foundation's criteria are entitled to carry the Fairtrade Mark, an independent guarantee of good practice.

Fair trade commodities include coffee, tea, cocoa, bananas, mangoes, honey, orange juice and sugar. Because of the complexity of setting prices (tea, for example, comes in so many quality grades it is impossible to set one price that suits all) there is no universal fair trade standard. Fair trade cannot eliminate all risk or bring benefits to all, but it is a growing market. With even Starbucks and Dunkin' Donuts selling fair trade coffee, the tentacles of ethical trading are reaching deeper into the world of the multinationals. The products are widely on offer; all it takes now is consumer commitment to transform the lives of millions of small producers.

The No Nonsense Guide
to Fair Trade
David Ranson
Verso Books 2001
ISBN 1-8598433-4-4

THE AMERICAN FOOTPRINT

if the whole world ate the way we do

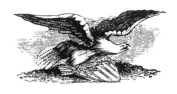

The average American is an obese American. National annual average consumption is 60 pounds of cakes and cookies, 23 gallons of ice cream, 7 pounds of potato chips, 200 sticks of gum, 576 cans of carbonated drinks, 90 pounds of fat, 134 pounds of refined sugar. That's just the average – those who eat still more of this nutritionally impoverished food are risking severe obesity.

America may be in the lead, but it is not alone. The fast food industry, among others, is determined to get the rest of the world to catch up. Apart from the nutrition problems thereby created, there are huge resource implications.

The amount of resources used by a person can be measured as an "ecological footprint," a term relating to the area of land used to provide a person's (or nation's) requirement for resources and to absorb their waste.

It takes an estimated ecological footprint of 24 acres of land to sustain an American.

National annual average consumption includes 60 pounds of cake and 23 gallons of ice cream

A Canadian needs 17 acres and an Italian gets by on nine. As a nation, the US has an ecological footprint that exceeds all of North and South America. Europe is not far behind.

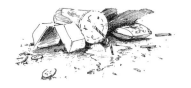

By comparison, the ecological footprint of an Indian is just under one acre.

It's not just land that's at stake. It takes 60 gallons of water to grow a pound of potatoes, 110 gallons to grow a pound of wheat and 12,500 gallons to produce a pound of beef.

It would take at least four Planet Earths to support the world's population on the American diet and

It would take at least four Earths to support the world's population on the American diet

lifestyle. Development that is based on increasing the income and consumption of the poorest 4.6 billion ignores the limits of the planet's resources. Stopping wasteful over-consumption is a far more effective way to stop the mining of the earth's natural capital. In America, the USDA Natural Resources Inventory calculates that 2.1 billion tons of soil were lost to wind and water erosion in 1992 alone. As Mark Twain famously remarked: "The problem with land is they stopped making it some time ago."

The world has 3.2 billion acres of cropland and 11.4 billion acres of grazing land. The World Widelife Fund estimates that we are already exceeding the carrying capacity of the earth by 30%, using up land and trees that are not being replaced, diminishing the stocks available for the increased world population of the future.

The waste from our over-consumption is a problem, too: CO2, sewage and packaging materials all need to be reduced or recycled. Cutting back on excessive food consumption, particularly of meat, would help to bring resource-use into balance, while reducing the obesity that brings ill health in its wake.

Societies that can reduce their ecological footprint may be the economic successes of the future. Those dependent on other nations' resources are in a precarious position. The US has to resort to the violent capture of global assets in order to maintain a lifestyle that is built around big cars and fast food. At the Earth Summit in Rio de Janeiro in 1992, George H. W. Bush announced: "The American way of life is not negotiable." As far as the rest of the world is concerned, the future of life on Earth is not negotiable. Herein lie the seeds of future conflict.

As we look towards a sustainable future, counting the number of heads will not be as important as measuring the size of the feet.

• The Soil Association in the UK estimates that a vegetarian family of four could be fed from three acres of land, or 3/4 acre (0.3 hectares) per person. A vegan family would eat well on even less without the need for livestock. These diets thus dramatically reduce a person's ecological footprint.

Our Ecological Footprint
Mathis Wackernagel, William Rees
New Society Publishers 1995
ISBN: 0-8657131-2-X

GOVERNMENT

calling the shots

"The freedom and happiness of man... are the sole objects of all legitimate government."
Thomas Jefferson

At times public interest is at odds with government policy. So, how optimistic can we be that government policy can ever help rather than hinder progress towards healthier food and farming?

Few will deny that capitalism operating in free markets with fair competition brings

Adam Smith warned in 1776 that larger businesses would attempt to harness the power of government

economic benefit to all sectors of society and rewards innovation. But Adam Smith warned in *Wealth of Nations*, way back in 1776, that larger businesses would inevitably attempt to harness the power of government to suppress smaller competitors to the detriment of overall prosperity. This seems to be what has happened to our food and farming.

In capitalism, wealth is measured as financial capital. That's how government does it too – it exists by taxing financial capital via income tax, corporation tax and sales taxes. But there are other forms of capital, "social capital" and "natural capital," that underpin financial prosperity and stability but are more difficult to value in a profit and loss statement.

Social capital is a village hall that has a different event on every evening and brings together the young, the old and the commuters. Voluntary organizations, cooperatives, clubs and societies build networks and support systems that lead to reduced crime, better health, care for the sick and elderly and greater trust between individuals. These efforts save government money – in health, welfare and employment.

Natural capital is the combined value of all the natural assets we enjoy: clean air, beautiful countryside and townscapes, fertile soil, unpolluted water. When we protect Natural Capital we can spend less on restoring damaged environments, cleaning up pollution and dealing with its health consequences.

Government's job is to create a balance between the creation of financial capital and the maintenance and nurturing of social and natural capital. When the pressure on government from financial interests leads to a reduction in social and natural capital then the economy as a whole is the loser. It's not just the national economy, either, we live in a globalized economy.

When the World Health Organization issued guidelines in April 2003 that stated that sugar should not form more than 10% of a person's diet, the US Sugar Association (including Coca-Cola, Pepsi and General Foods) went on the offensive. They threatened to get Congress to withdraw funding from the WHO unless they withdrew their sugar recommendations and instead recommended that sugar could comfortably form 25% of a person's diet.

The Food and Drug Administration (FDA) is the government body which regulates and polices industry that represents 25% of the total US economy: food, drink and drugs. It exercises its power over drugs through 18 "Expert Committees" that are composed of members

54% of FDA committee experts have links with drug companies

who are bound by a rule that they cannot have an obvious financial conflict of interest. Yet 54% of the experts on these committees have direct links with drug companies that stand to benefit from the FDA's regulatory decisions. How so? The FDA is allowed to issue a waiver of the conflict of interest rules if they believe an expert can bring valuable knowledge to the committee. These are the people who decide which drugs are prescribed in the USA and which are not. The FDA vigorously attacks the importation of cheaper medication, providing a profit protection scheme that underpins the huge profitability of drugs sold in the USA, often selling at four to five times the price for identical medicines in Europe.

What's the answer? Not permitting waivers of the rules on the composition of the Expert Committees? If the FDA were an independent, non-governmental body that simply made recommendations based on trust that it had earned and had no enforcement powers, then doctors and consumers could decide in a free market for medicines and information about them. There would be no opportunities for potential corruption.

In 1993, with FDA approval, Monsanto launched Posilac, (or rBGH:recombinant Bovine Growth Hormone) that increases a cow's

> With an independent FDA with no enforcement powers, doctors could pick drugs in a free market

milk output and extends its lactation period by three months. Canada refused to permit Posilac, against a background of allegations that they were offered bribes by Monsanto and complaints about harassment by their scientists. No European country will permit its use, because of human health concerns, particularly in respect of prostate cancer. The FDA refused an application under the Freedom of Information Act for a copy of an FDA study on Posilac on the grounds that, if the public learned the results, it would "irreparably harm" Monsanto. Margaret Miller, who put the original Posilac approval application to the FDA in 1989 then left Monsanto to work for the FDA. Her first job at the FDA was to decide whether to approve Monsanto's application. (By 2004 sales of Posilac were in steep decline – government support still can't overcome producer and consumer resistance.)

Industry, as Adam Smith foresaw, lobbies constantly in government to bend policy in its direction, whether agribusiness, military equipment or pharmaceuticals. Small companies and industries have no such lobbying power, consumers even less. However, organizations such as the Sierra Club, Greenpeace or the Center for Science in the Public Interest can sway policy towards the protection of natural and social capital. As these pressure groups become stronger and make alliances at home and abroad with counterpart organizations they can form an effective counterbalance to narrow industrial interests.

In *Uncommon Sense,* Gregory Sams argues that, if insurance companies governed the world, there would be no nuclear power, no genetic engineering and no global warming. Simple – nobody can do business without insurance and insurance companies don't tolerate unfathomable or extreme risks. (It was pressure from insurance companies on government that brought in mandatory seatbelts and other road safety measures.) But insurance companies don't run the world and nuclear power and genetic engineering are authorized by governments that exempt the participants from liability and the victims from compensation.

Government responds to market situations and organized political pressure. So does business. We can't do without government or business, so we must make policy work to ensure the optimal balance between social, natural and financial capital. We can do this by actively supporting organizations that influence policy to make our food and farming better for us, for our children, farming families, rural communities and the natural environment. We can apply pressure on the food industry by buying safe and nutritious food. "The hinge that squeaks loudest gets the most oil." Squeaking loudly – through organizations, as individuals and through a free press – is the way to persuade government to ensure that social and natural capital are not sacrificed for narrow, short-term financial gain.

"Freedom and liberty lose out by default because good people are not vigilant."
Archbishop Desmond Tutu

"It is not our purpose to endanger the financial interest of the pharmaceutical companies."
FDA Commissioner Dr. Charles C. Edwards

Uncommon Sense
Gregory Sams
Chaos Works 1998
ISBN 0-9531301-0-X

The Captive State
George Monbiot
Macmillan 2000
ISBN 0-3339016-4-9

THE FARMER FEEDS THEM ALL

the family farm's importance to our culture

Should farmers have a union? It makes sense for farmworkers, but it is strange to see landowners, the epitome of independent property-owning enterprise, operating a union.

It was Thomas Jefferson who believed that the foundations of a stable democracy stood with broadly distributed property wealth and insisted that farmland, ideally 40-acre parcels, should belong to the family that worked it and not to landlords or real estate companies. He

Thomas Jefferson believed that farms should belong to the families who worked them, not landlords

saw the small landholder as the moral soul of the nation, self-sufficient and at the core of a healthy body politic. His political rival, Alexander Hamilton, saw an America in which manufacturing would dominate and he helped frame the alliance that eventually emerged between government and business.

Between 1940 and 1998 the following changes took place:

- Average farm size: grew from 135 acres to 469 acres
- Number of farms: fell from 6.1 million to 2 million
- Farming population: fell from 31 million to 3 million
- Net farm income $59 billion (in '98 dollars) down to $55 billion

Small farms are more productive than large farms, but lobbying by vertically integrated agribusiness corporations has reinforced a trend towards giant hog farms, cattle feedlots and intensive chicken units. Agribusiness corporations, with subsidized production of ethanol and corn syrup and with monopoly control over pricing, ensure that family farmers are marginally profitable while they benefit hugely. The Cato Institute calculates that 43% of ADM's annual profits are from products such as corn syrup and ethanol that the US government subsidizes. Small farms are diverse, they "multi-task" and produce vegetables and specialty foods. Their meat animals are less likely to carry pathogenic bacteria. They pollute less and connect with local communities. As income has fallen, farming communities have moved from healthy, middle-class environments to rural ghettoes, with unemployment, violence and despair – the heartland has become America's Third World. Independent farmers are a tiny minority and no longer have the political power that they enjoyed in the 19th and early 20th century.

So how can they plead their case? Who speaks for the family farmer in the corridors of power?

The American Farm Bureau calls itself the "Voice of Agriculture." It was founded in 1919 by representatives from 30 farming states, but it quickly became a lobby for agribusiness and the promotion of corporate farming. Its main income is derived from its role as an insurance company and its 4.9 million membership derives from the requirement that you have to join in order to purchase insurance. The Farm Bureau actively supports the industrialization of agriculture. "Big is not necessarily bad," in the words of Farm Bureau President Bob Stallman,

Farming communities have moved from healthy middle-class environments to rural ghettoes with unemployment and violence

while defending the concentration of agriculture during a House Agriculture Committee hearing in July 2000.

The National Grange, founded in 1867, now has 300,000 members who really are farmers and has a democratic structure spreading through 3600 communities in 37 states. Its HQ building in Washington, D.C. serves as a focal point. Grange policy is established at grass-roots level where members set out their "issues of concern" that are then represented to policymakers in the capital. Its vision is somewhat defensive: to stem the loss of members (difficult when farmers are going out of business), to be a relevant organization with effective leaders and "reducing resistance to change." In practice, they lobby for cheaper prescription drugs, better telecommunications in rural areas and support for biofuels.

More politically edgy is the National Farmers Union, with 250,000 farmer and rancher members, founded in 1902. It is committed to turning around the concentration of monopolistic power in production, processing

> The National Farmers Union is committed to turning around monopolistic power in production

and retail, to bringing youth into farming and to bringing in real fair trade that will strengthen farmers' negotiating power. They sponsored legislation to allow farmers to save patented seed for re-use and they monitor the farmer's share of the food dollar (Wheaties $3.49 – farmer share 5¢). Their involvement with

the International Federation of Agricultural Producers (IFAP) reflects the need for farmers to form global alliances if they are to be able to balance the oligopoly power of the big agribusiness empires. IFAP represents 500 million family farms in 70 countries. Together their strength may bring some hope for the future of family farmers, the true individualists of free-enterprise democracies, but the multinationals will not give up their share of the consumer's food dollar without a fight.

Organic farmers, a growing minority within a declining sector, have a stronger influence on policy because of the support they receive from environmental, health and wildlife organizations who realize that organic farming delivers on many of their aspirations. Organic processors, retailers and consumers respect and value the culture of the family farm and the values it represents, elevating the producer's status and putting a dollar value on that respect by paying a fair price for organic produce. Market forces, for the organic farmer, have been a blessing rather than curse.

The comment that "farming is a business, just like any other" doesn't ring true, and, as people understand the importance of agriculture to a nation's culture, a revaluation of farming's important social role is emerging.

THE FARMER FEEDS US ALL
You may talk of all the nobles of the earth,
Of the kings who hold the nations in their thrall,
Yet in this we all agree, if we only look and see,
That the farmer is the man that feeds us all.

Words and Music by
Knowles Shaw (1834-1878)

PESTICIDES

there's no escape

From planting to harvest, crops are attractive to seed-eating, sap-sucking, leaf-eating, root-nibbling pests. So we "zap" them. Weeds grow vigorously when their surrounding crops are fed with artificial fertilizers. So we "zap" them, too. Natural methods can protect crops, but poison is the cheapest solution. However, pesticidal poison is indiscriminate and its cheapness conceals an unpaid cost to society and the environment.

The World Health Organization (WHO) estimates there are 500,000 pesticide-related

> Pesticides attack biodiversity, leading to loss of wildlife and the disappearance of species

poisonings per year including 5,000 accidental deaths. The US Environment Protection Agency calculates that between 10,000 and 20,000 cases of pesticide poisoning incidents occur among US agricultural workers each year.

But that's just the tip of the iceberg. Pesticides attack biodiversity, leading to loss of wildlife and the disappearance – forever – of species. But pesticides have other talents. They can be:

Carcinogenic – causing cancer

Mutagenic – causing or increasing frequency of mutation

Teratogenic – damaging to an embryo or fetus

Fattening – when the liver cannot dispose of poisons they can be wrapped in fat and stored for later attention, i.e. as cellulite. (This is one reason why dieters often feel ill as shedding fat also entails pesticides re-entering the system.)

Endocrine-disruptors – some pesticide molecules are similar to human hormones such as estrogen, so the body's hormone balance becomes confused and upset (see chapter "Estrogen").

Many of the worst pesticides, such as DDT insecticide and Atrazine herbicide, have been banned or restricted in much of the industrial world. Nonetheless, these chemicals continue to be used in poorer countries, giving rise to an unfortunate paradox. When a farmer in the tropics sprays his crops, some pesticides are carried up by evaporation into the rain clouds. Some rise into the stratosphere, where they are carried around the planet only to be re-released when the clouds pass over the colder polar regions, condense and fall as rain or snow. This is why Scandinavian countries have, ironically, such high levels of DDT in their environment and food, despite banning the chemicals in the 1960s. It is also responsible for childhood cancers and sexual deformity among the Inuit children of Canada because Arctic foods such as caribou, cod and berry fruits have high levels of residues.

In Britain, all known sources of spring water still contain traces of the gender-changing, hormone-disruptor atrazine, despite its use being restricted in the early 1990s.

Other chemical use persists. A 2001 report by Britain's Pesticides Residues Committee revealed levels of Dicofol (a DDT derivative) in strawberries at 10 times the maximum residue level (MRL). Dicofol use in Florida causes genital shrinkage in male alligators. It makes reproduction impossible. The report also showed higher pesticide residues in wholegrain (non-organic) bread than in white bread and

British spring water still contains traces of a hormone disruptor

that farmed salmon always contains significant levels of organochlorine pesticides (used to control sea lice).

High-fiber bran cereals, lettuces, citrus fruit and apples also showed multiple pesticide residues at levels that raised concerns about the "cocktail effect." This means that three pesticides consumed together can have 100 times the damaging effect of each one eaten separately. The maximum permitted residue level for pesticides is set at 1/100th of the level at which tests have shown them to be harmful, so the accumulative effect of a cocktail of pesticides quickly negates individual safety margins set by regulators. Where crops are sprayed with as many as 36 different pesticides, some of them systemic, washing or peeling is useless. In an apparently healthy meal that includes salmon, whole wheat bread, carrots, lettuce, apples and strawberries one could easily be consuming more than 100 pesticides. All this adds to the exposure to synthetic chemicals in bodycare and household products, plus the inhalation of airborne by-products of diesel and gasoline engines.

Another pesticide-related phenomenon is more apparent. "Pesticide suicides" in India are estimated at 20,000 per annum. Farmers using pesticides find that pests develop resistance. So, more agrichemicals are needed and soil

If pesticides were stained blue so that residues showed up in food, who would buy it?

fertility declines. Eventually the whole process becomes unsustainable and the farmer is faced with leaving his land. Or he swallows enough pesticides to escape these problems – forever.

How can farmers reduce pesticide residues? Many pesticides are applied on a "just-in-case" basis to prevent cosmetic damage by insects. For example, unripe apricots are sprayed to avoid insect damage that puts "freckles" on the fruit. Hothouse plants such as lettuces, cucumbers and tomatoes are routinely sprayed against whitefly and red spider mite. But there are alternatives. Chemical-free methods include crop rotation, release of natural predator populations, traps, beetle banks and physical barriers. "Companion planting" is a system where plants that repel certain pests are planted alongside those that don't. All these techniques are less than 100% effective, so that you may find that the edge of a leaf has been nibbled or that there is an aphid lurking inside a lettuce leaf. However, the invisible risks from pesticides tip the balance, for many people, in favor of organic food. If pesticides were stained bright blue so that residues showed up in food, who would buy blue fruit and vegetables?

Biopesticides: *Bacillus thuringiensis* (Bt), a bacterium that kills insects, has been used successfully by organic farmers since the 1960s. It disappears three days after application and leaves no residues. However, its toxic secretion has now been engineered into patented biotech crops such as Bt maize. Insect resistance is already developing due to the continuous exposure of the permanently "on" genetic modification and the persistent presence of Bt toxin in soil. An important tool of organic farming thus risks being lost.

• A Cuban biopesticide, Griselef, based on spores of *Bacillus sphericus*, is specific to mosquito species which feed on blood. It only needs spraying one to three times to wipe out a mosquito population, compared to 40-50 sprayings needed for Fenthion (an organopesticide that has replaced DDT). It is cheap and effective and, most important, causes no harm to humans, animals and other insects, just malaria-spreading mosquitoes.

• Most parks, sports fields and golf courses are sprayed with pesticides regularly. Few of them post notices or cordon off sprayed areas.

• Sampling by the Centers for Disease Control found residues of 15 different pesticides in urine samples from men in rural Missouri and Minneapolis. The pesticides came primarily from drinking water. The researchers found that, the higher the level of pesticide residues the men had, the lower was the quantity and viability of their sperm. In the United States, where 15% of the population obtains their water from their own wells, cisterns or springs, the EPA advises that water should be checked for pesticides. Filtration systems make sense — pesticide levels can fluctuate depending on when farmers spray — peaks of pollution may not be detected by routine testing.

Pesticide Action Network
North America
www.panna.org

ENERGY

it's exhausting

Fossil fuels are running out. The need for alternative sources of energy is urgent. "Energy crops" are a hoped-for new market for agriculture and their story highlights much of what has gone wrong with modern agriculture.

In Germany, "bio-diesel" blends use up surplus subsidized rapeseed oil by mixing it with diesel

> Cornell University estimates it takes 1.7 gallons of fossil fuels to make 1 gallon of ethanol

fuel for use by public service vehicles. In the US, oil companies supply "gasohol" which is a blend of 90% gasoline and 10% ethanol – alcohol distilled from corn. Some have gone further and offer EP85, a blend of 85% ethanol mixed with 15% gasoline. Although ethanol is more expensive, government tax breaks and allowances mean EP85 can be sold at the same price as gasoline.

The National Corn Growers' Association boasts that over 5% of US corn production in 2002 went to ethanol production. That's over three million acres of farmland devoted to reducing the use of fossil fuels. Or is it?

An acre of corn yields 328 gallons of ethanol. But that corn is grown using agricultural machinery, artificial fertilizers, pesticides and herbicides – all using fossil fuels. Converting it into a fermented mash and distilling it to produce ethanol uses yet more energy.

Cornell University estimates that it thus takes 1.7 gallons of fossil fuels to make one gallon of ethanol. The actual cost of corn ethanol is $1.74 per gallon, compared to $0.95 for gasoline. Tax breaks and subsidies make it competitive – at a cost to the taxpayer of more than $1 billion per year. Even if the corn were free, and then converted to ethanol, it still wouldn't be competitive in the marketplace. (Ethanol could be made directly from fossil fuels for $0.95 per gallon, but the tax rebate only applies to ethanol made from corn or other biomass.)

It's not just fossil fuels that are wasted producing ethanol. Growing corn erodes soil 12 times faster than it can be reformed, leading to large-scale topsoil loss. Irrigated corn uses groundwater at a rate 25 times faster than the underground reservoirs are filling up and leads to salinization. Topsoil loss and salinization are why 1% of the world's arable land is going out of production every year. All this waste and yet ethanol is sold as an "ecological" fuel. If every American drove an ethanol-powered vehicle the entire land area of the US would have to be given over to corn production for fuel.

So why is gasohol being pushed so hard? As long as corn is subsidized more fertilizers, herbicides, GM seeds, pesticides and agricultural machinery can be sold. Rather than burning crop surpluses in the petrol tank, the land could be put into "retirement," and soil fertility rebuilt. But there's nothing to show for that in the next quarter's profit and loss accounts. Archer Daniels Midland (ADM) lobbies intensively to ensure the US government keeps up the subsidies on ethanol. ADM produces more than 50% of all ethanol used as fuel.

In the debate about genetic engineering the recurrent refrain of GM supporters is: "The

There's plenty of existing capacity to feed the world

world's population will soon reach 10 billion – without GM crops we won't be able to feed the world." Thirty one million acres of land are already out of production in the US under the Conservation Reserve Program; three million are devoted to producing corn ethanol. An estimated further 15 million acres produce corn that is converted expensively into corn syrup by ADM, with generous government subsidies. There's plenty of existing capacity to feed the world.

But there's a further argument for gasohol: it reduces America's dependency on fossil fuels from politically volatile areas such as the Middle East and Venezuela. "We don't need military expenditure to protect the corn fields of the Midwest," claim ethanol's proponents. But as ethanol production is based on an increased need for fossil fuels the reverse is actually true.

Intensive agriculture takes 12 calories' worth of fossil fuels to produce one calorie of food. If oil prices rise the economics of agriculture change. With oil above $40 per barrel, intensive agriculture can no longer

The taxpayer's interest has been subverted by agribusiness' control of the political process

compete with low-input alternatives such as organic farming, which use 50% less energy to produce the same output. The bio-fuels, too, would become even more expensive.

Fuel cells, solar power and other "alternative" electricity generating systems will become more, rather than less, competitive as oil prices rise. However, the agribusiness and the oil lobbies continue to make them less-favored options. The wasteful use of finite resources illustrates how the consumer/taxpayer's interest has been subverted by agribusiness' control of the political process.

• Germany's "Bio-diesel" is a blend of diesel oil with either rapeseed or soy oil, or animal fats such as lard or butter. The economics are, like those of petrol, dependent on subsidies to compensate for the cost differentials. It would be cheaper to buy the crops and throw them in the sea.

Food, Energy and Society
David Pimentel, Marcia Pimentel
Colorado University Press 1996
ISBN 0-8708138-6-2

ORGANOPHOSPHATES

the poison hierarchy

Before hormone usage the earliest growth promoters used in intensive animal production were organophosphates, where very low doses were enough to increase fat development. However, organophosphates, which are a "broad-pectrum" class of insecticides, have known toxic effects on the nervous system. Large doses were used in the gas chambers at Auschwitz and were also tested for use as nerve gas in warfare.

Before considering organophosphates we have to look back at organochlorines. These were the first and least safe generation of pesticides that included DDT, Lindane, aldrin and dieldrin. All are persistent and accumulate in the food chain. Lindane, the last of the organochlorines still being used, was phased out in Europe in 2002 and is also banned in California, though permitted in the rest of the US. It is commonly used in developing countries, particularly on cocoa trees. It was, however, the clear association with increased risk of breast cancer that led, after much resistance from farmers and chemical companies, to the EU ban. The ban has encouraged farmers to look to other chemicals.

Organophosphates are claimed to be safer than the organochlorines, but evidence is emerging that they may be just as bad – in a different way. Their use during World War II should tell us something. As a nerve gas, they slow the

Organophosphates were used as nerve gas in World War II

transmission of nerve impulses, causing nervous system and brain failure.

So why use it on cattle?

When organophosphates are consumed, they restrict the conversion of fats, held in reserve, back into glucose. Instead, the fat just accumulates. They damage nerves, weaken muscle fibers and reduce the desire to exercise – which helps produce tender, fatty meat. The use of organophosphates as growth promoters in cattle has finally been banned in agriculture, because of their toxic side effects.

In Britain, phosmet, a blend of a thalidomide compound and an organophosphate, is rubbed on the spines of cattle to get rid of warble fly larvae. From the spine, phosmet can penetrate to all parts of the cow's body, killing the infestation. Mark Purdey, a researcher in Somerset, argues that "mad cow disease"

The use of organophosphates as growth promoters in cattle has finally been banned

could initiate from this practice. A fetal calf's head is positioned directly beneath the mother's spine, so could receive a direct dose of organophosphates at a crucial stage in the development of its nervous system. Phosmet is occasionally used for lice control in the United States and mad cow disease has been rare.

Organophosphates are also still widely used on vegetable and fruit crops. In February 2004, a Cancer Prevention Research Program study found organophosphate residues in the urine of adult farmworkers and their children, as well as in their house dust. In January 1998 an Environmental Working Group study found organophosphates at unsafe levels in apples, pears and grapes, in some cases exceeding federal safety standards by 10 times or more.

Organophosphates are used in head lice lotions and creams for children. For years cosmetic and bodycare manufacturers have pooh-poohed the idea that the chemicals in their products could get into the bloodstream. That was before nicotine patches. It is now known that up to 60% of what you put on your skin can enter your bloodstream. Unlike ingestion by mouth, where a substance has to pass through the defenses of saliva, hydrochloric acid in the stomach and the protective flora of the digestive system, substances rubbed on the skin penetrate quickly and effectively. A study in 1997 by Britain's Health & Safety Executive and Dr. Vyvyan Howard of Liverpool University established that the organophosphate in head lice solutions could put children five times over government safety limits and that repeated use may damage the nervous system. It is even thought that Creutzfeldt-Jakob Disease could arise from head lice treatments. Alzheimer's disease symptoms closely mirror those of organophosphate poisoning.

Monsanto's Roundup herbicide may not be as immediately harmful as other organophosphates, but the intensive lobbying by Monsanto that led to the 200-fold increase in Maximum Residue Level for Roundup does mean considerable increased exposure. Roundup also contains 25% polyacrylamide, which helps it stick evenly to plants. At high temperatures polyacrylamide breaks down into acrylamide, a strong carcinogen that has been found in potato chips, crispbreads, French fries and other foods cooked at high temperatures.

Organophosphates are also used in sheep dips, flea treatments for pets, wood treatment, garden pesticides and as additives in gasoline, aviation fuel, lubricating oils and flame-retardant treatments.

Over-exposure to organophosphates produces what doctors call SLUD: Salivation, Lacrimation (tears), Urination, Defecation. This leads to paralysis, confusion and convulsions ending in death by central respiratory failure. Lower level exposure has been connected with damage to the nervous system, depression, cardiac problems and eye defects.

Organophosphates will probably, one day, be phased out as the evidence of their harm becomes overwhelming. Even the "Five-A-Day" campaign to encourage people to eat more fruit and vegetables may suffer from consumer anxiety to avoid organophosphates. Cutting vegetables out of the diet, however, may be worse to health than consuming some residues. But if you regularly consume fruit and vegetables, it makes sense to avoid organophosphate residues. The obvious answer is to eat organic produce.

The Detox Diet
Paula Baillie-Hamilton
Michael Joseph 2002
ISBN 0-7181454-5-3

Pesticides Action Network North America
www.panna.org

http://ist-socrates.berkeley.edu/~jmp
/alex-html.html

ESTROGEN

the feminizing hormone

Most of us think of hormones, estrogen for example, as natural substances that circulate in our bodies and affect behavior and body cycles. Most of, however, don't know the full story.

The use of hormones in the production of meat really took off in the '60s. A synthetic version of the feminizing hormone estrogen, Diethylstilbestrol (DES), was heralded as a "wonder drug" to beef feedlot farmers who inserted a hormone implant behind the ear of a heifer or steer to increase its weight – and their profit. DES also produced a fattier, more "well-marbled" meat that made for juicier steaks. There were concerns about the risks to humans of consuming DES and farmers were told to remove the implant five days before slaughter to allow estrogen levels in the meat to drop. Few farmers did so, as removal of the implant led to immediate weight (and profit) loss.

DES was also prescribed to women who had miscarriages to reduce the risk of miscarrying again. The supporting research, however, was flawed; miscarriages actually increased with DES and it was banned when it was found to increase the risk of breast cancer too. Worse, it led to an even greater risk of breast cancer in the daughters of women who took DES because of excessive estrogen during pregnancy. Worse still was the risk of breast cancer in their granddaughters. All the eggs a woman will ever produce are created in the fetal stage of her own development. So, the egg that produces the granddaughter was created by the grandmother. Effects can increase from generation to generation.

The discovery of the harmful effects of DES led to a call for a ban on its use as a growth promoter. This was fiercely resisted by farmers but by the 1980s both the US and EU had placed a ban.

A black market flourished among farmers and illicit DES use continues, particularly in Southeast Asia, Latin America and Eastern Europe.

In the EU there is now, after years of pressure, an outright ban on the use of all hormones in meat production. In the US, however, other feminizing hormones have been substituted for DES. To boost their effectiveness, they are combined with masculinizing hormones – anabolic steroids – so that the animal goes through phases of fatty tissue development as the feminizing hormones dominate, followed by rapid muscle growth as the anabolic steroids kick in, followed by more estrogen-led fatty tissue development. The result is increased meat yield.

To protect such production methods, by the early 1990s over 20 states in the US had passed "Agricultural Slander Acts" making it a criminal offense to criticize agricultural practices without indisputable scientific evidence. Fines can also be charged equal to the value of the estimated loss of sales suffered as a result of any "slanders." Without independent research and with the possibility that a court might side with scientists representing the hormone industry, there has been a reluctance to speak out.

At the World Trade Organization, the US went on to accuse the EU of putting up trade barriers by banning the import of hormone-enhanced American beef. The EU, anxious to protect its food exports to the US, but unwilling to compromise the health and sexuality of its citizens, made a concession: they agreed to allow the import of US beef as long as it was labelled as produced with growth hormones. European consumers could then make an informed choice.

The WTO fined the EU $120 million for opposing hormones

Not good enough, said the US; there's no risk so there should be no labeling. The WTO agreed, and in 2001 the EU was fined $120 million, payable every year, for fighting to keep hormones off Europeans' plates.

There are, however, other sources of hormones known as "xen-estrogens," or "estrogen-mimics." In 2001, biologists discovered that 84% of female salmon in the Columbia River in Washington were born males and changed sex by the time they reached maturity. The cause is believed to be "estrogen mimicry" from industrial chemicals and herbicides.

The molecular structure of most herbicides is remarkably similar to that of the estrogen molecule. When a herbicide molecule is consumed, it finds its way to the hormone receptors that are tailored to fit with estrogen and its identity is mistaken. The body sometimes is confused into thinking that estrogen levels are too high and stops the production of natural estrogen, which can lead to masculinization in females. At other times the estrogen mimic activates femininity, with the possible effects of enlarged breasts in a male or female, or reduced testicle size in a male. Similarly, the presence of estrogens and xenestrogens increases the level of the male hormone testosterone. This breaks down into the chemical dihydrotestosterone, the main cause of prostate enlargement and cancer. There has been a greatly increased level of breast cancer in the late 20th century and testicular cancer is now the biggest cancer threat to 20-34 year-old males.

• "It is conservatively estimated that most people have measurable quantities of between 300 and 500 chemicals in their bodies, which have been introduced to the planet within the last 50 years and would not have been present prior to that... It is generally agreed that fetal and infant life are the most susceptible periods for the action of hormone disrupting chemicals to have their maximum adverse effects."
Dr. Vyvyan Howard

• In East Anglia, where intensive agriculture leaves high levels of herbicide spray drifting in the air and residues in the water supply, a woman's risk of developing breast cancer has reached 40%.

• In Denmark, the sperm count among organic farmers is double that of conventional farmers, possibly because of reduced exposure to herbicides and their estrogenic effect.

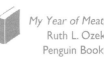

My Year of Meat
Ruth L. Ozeki
Penguin Books
ISBN: 0-1402804-6-

GENETICALLY MODIFIED FOOD

but can we eat it?

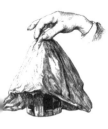

The patenting of discoveries about life is a new development. Thus far, patenting has been restricted to innovation and invention. However, the existence of Genetically Modified Organisms (GMOs) is now a reality and for most people the primary concern is "Are GMOs and food containing them safe to eat?"

In 1993, 11 out of 17 scientists at the US Food and Drug Administration opposed the approval of the first GM tomato variety because of concerns about its safety after feeding trials. However, they were overruled by their bosses, who were under great political pressure to grant approval. At the same time, the FDA established a principle of "substantial equivalence," which stated that GM foods would no longer have to undergo safety testing because there was no significant difference between them and non-GM foods. It is this principle, which the US seeks to apply worldwide through WTO negotiations, that is at the heart of the debate about GM foods and safety. It is why the USDA

The US seeks to have the WTO ban GM labeling worldwide

opposes labeling of GM food – arguing that to give consumers a choice implies that something is wrong with the GM option.

Although it is often claimed that GM foods are the most heavily tested in the history of the food industry, there have only ever been ten scientific feeding safety trials using GM food, five of which (the independent ones) showed differences that were the cause of concern. Nor can we look to the manufacturers to take responsibility for safety. The corporate attitude is summed up by the comments of Phil Angell, Monsanto's Director of Corporate Communications: "Monsanto should not have to vouchsafe the safety of biotech (GM) food. Our interest is in selling as much of it as possible. Assuring its safety is the FDA's job."

The feeding trials that have been carried out are not encouraging. Dr. Arpad Pusztai's

Every independent study has shown cause for concern with genetically modified food

research in 1998 showed that rats fed on GM potatoes developed intestinal lesions, or "leaky gut" – similar to the results found with feeding trials using GM Flavr-Savr tomatoes in 1993. Ulcerative colitis, Crohn's disease, autism, malabsorption syndrome, food allergies and eczema are just a few of the diseases associated with leaky gut. Pusztai was forced to resign but when the research was published, the Royal Society, Britain's national academy of science, called for further investigation. Unsurprisingly, no scientist has dared take up the challenge and no biotech company has offered to fund such research.

In 2001 the British Medical Association report into GMOs claimed "insufficient evidence" to inform a decision on their safety.

In May 2002, 17 pig breeders in Iowa reported a sharp decline, up to 80%, in the conception rate of breeding sows. All had one thing in common: they had only used their own farm-grown, genetically modified Bt maize in their pig feed. Iowa farmer Jerry Rosman commented: "We're working with a problem that no one has ever heard of before." The maize had unusually high levels of fusarium, a mould associated with fungal poisons known as mycotoxins known to cause pseudo-pregnancy. This was a new and unknown mycotoxin that had emerged in reaction to the engineered toxin in the GM maize. The Iowa Farm Bureau recommended that farmers who breed their own pigs stop using GM corn. Humans who eat corn products were given no such warning.

In October 2000, after careful research into the matter, Munich RE and Swiss RE, the world's leading reinsurers, announced that they would not insure farmers or food processors for any liability arising from GM foods or farming. Since GM crops were now virtually uninsurable, the EU Commission and industry lobbyists pressured the European Parliament to put GM food producers beyond the normal laws of liability. (Much the same happened in the nuclear-power business; it was – and is – uninsurable. Governments have had to promise to cover the costs of accidents.)

The companies that own the patents and have a financial interest in promoting GMO use do most of the research into GM crops that secures their approval. Differences occur in test results between independent researchers and those with a commercial interest. The biotech industry, for example, claims precision in the insertion of genes as a surety of GMO safety. Such claims, however, are undermined by the discovery that, while the human genome contains 30,000 genes, 250,000 different proteins are produced in the body. This means that many genes are multi-functional, with many functions that we don't yet understand. It isn't surprising that

unforeseen consequences of gene transfer have been found in plants – deformed cotton bolls, woody stems in soy beans, breeding problems

Only extensive feeding trials can really assess the safety of GM food

in sows. Only extensive feeding trials can really assess the safety of GM foods. They should be long-term trials – humans who eat GM food can live for 70 years or so, the average feeding trial lasts 28-45 days.

Another argument put forward for the safety of GM foods is that Americans have been eating them since 1997 with no ill effects. However, food-related illnesses in the US are estimated to have doubled since 1997 and the accidental entry into the food chain, in 2001, of Aventis' modified Starlink maize led to many complaints of allergic reaction. Three years later, Starlink genes are still appearing in other varieties of corn – these things don't go away. With the advent of "pharming" – the growing of GM pharmaceutical crops – we face the possibility of permanent contamination of our food supply with self-replicating drugs.

GM food provides no real benefit to farmers. US farm subsidies have gone from $3 billion to $150 billion a year since GM crops were introduced. There are no nutritional benefits to GM food. The little safety testing there is indicates health risks. (Even the companies that sell GM seed are unhealthy. Calgene, who developed the Flavr-Savr tomato, went bankrupt and was bought by Monsanto, who ran out of money and was bought by Pharmacia Upjohn, who couldn't sell it, so gave its shares away to their shareholders). They want a total monopoly and to deny consumers freedom of choice. Without

> GM companies want a total monopoly and to deny consumers freedom of choice

that, the GM juggernaut may stop where it is. Meanwhile, GMOs are out there and questions about health risks remain unanswered.

• Plants such as maize, soybeans and oilseed rape are engineered to have herbicide resistance. This allows weed killer, such as the herbicide glufosinate, to be sprayed right up to harvest, greatly increasing the risk of residues in the final crop. Glufosinate is both a neurotoxin and a teratogen (causes embryo damage). Would these residues not seriously concern the biotech industry and our governments? Well before the introduction of GM crops, the biotech industry persuaded US and EU governments to increase the permitted residue of weed killers in foods to 20,000 times the previous level.

• Soybeans with engineered Brazil-nut protein were never put on the market because of the risk of fatal anaphylactic shock in nut-allergic consumers of "nut-free" products like soymilk.

• When GM canola protein was fed to chickens, their death rate was twice that of chickens fed non-GM protein.

*How to Avoid GM Food:
Hundreds of Brands, Products
and Ingredients to Avoid*
Joanna Blythman
Trafalgar Square 1999
ISBN: 1-8411518-7-4

FISHING FOR FOOD

fishy business

Fish is good for us, but we are not good for fish. An abundant and valuable source of nutritious food is disappearing because of wasteful over-fishing and pollution of the sea.

Fish is a source of protein and essential fatty acids and is also rich in iodine, necessary for the production of the thyroid hormone thyroxine, which regulates our energy levels (see chapter "Brain Food").

When the Grand Banks of Newfoundland were discovered in 1501 by Portuguese fishermen, they dropped baskets off the sides of their boats and lifted them out filled with cod. Ideal feeding and spawning conditions ensured a prolific supply of fish – until the late 1980s when cod stocks collapsed and the Canadian government banned their fishing until levels recovered. The recovery has been far slower than expected. One reason for this is that cod don't reproduce until they are six years old and smaller fish fall victim to predators. The Canadian government may have acted too late.

Deprived of fishing rights on the Grand Banks, European fishermen have sought fish elsewhere. The western coast of Africa provides rich fishing, and EU agreements with Mauritania and Senegal, burdened by debt and the need for foreign exchange, have opened up new fishing grounds inside their territorial waters. As the larger fish disappear the trawlers fish for smaller fish, often throwing back 80% to 90% of the "by-catch" that are not wanted or converting them to fishmeal for sale to European fish farms. Senegalese and Mauritanian fishermen, who fish in small wooden boats intended for inshore use, have to go further out to sea in search of fish. Many never return. Others abandon fishing and migrate to Europe, where, ironically, they may find work on large trawlers fishing in their native waters. Fish and rice, a traditional dish and the source of 75% of Senegalese protein intake, has become a scarce luxury. The world fish catch is worth $100 billion, government subsidies to fishermen are worth $20 billion annually. Subsidies enable fishermen to exhaust otherwise unprofitable declining fisheries. The "Friends of Fish" (New Zealand, Australia, Iceland, Peru, Chile, Philippines and the US) want such subsidies to end. The EU agrees, but wants to switch subsidies to helping fishermen to scrap excess fishing boats and find other employment. Japan

> Persistent organic pollutants build up in fish, particularly in oily fish and in fish livers

dismisses all such concerns as unfounded – it has higher subsidies to the fishing industry than the US and EU combined.

How safe is fish?

Persistent organic pollutants such as dioxin and polychlorinated biphenyls (PCBs) from industrial waste, ship paints, insulation and pesticides, build up in fish, particularly in oily fish and in fish livers. The manufacturers of fish oil capsules have found it difficult to keep within maximum residue level limits. Indeed cod liver oil can have high levels of dioxins. These and other pollutants find their way up the food chain to fish. As a result it may be best to eat fish only twice a week, enough to obtain the nutritional benefits without accumulating too many pollutants.

What about farming fish?

Aquaculture, or fish farming, is held out as the answer to the decline in wild fish stocks. However, it has problems of its own. A farmed salmon that escapes, may breed with a wild salmon, destroying the latter's genetic integrity. Antibiotics are used routinely to suppress disease and alleviate stress. Ivermectin, for example, is added to fish-feed to control sea lice, and organophosphates are poured over the salmon too. PCBs in farmed salmon tested by the EPA were 16 times the level in wild fish.

It takes 6 1/2 to 11 pounds of wild fish to make enough feed to produce one pound of farmed salmon.

Farmed salmon has higher fat content than wild salmon, but a lower content of the DHA and EPA essential fatty acids that make it nutritious. In blind taste-tests farmed salmon loses every time. The seabed beneath salmon cages takes years to recover from the pollution of excreta, drugs and pesticides used in the cages. The problem isn't confined to salmon. Sand eels, a vital component of a cod's diets in spring and early summer, are vacuumed up by Danish trawlers and then converted into fish oil and fishmeal, contributing to the fall in wild cod stocks.

Fish farmers say the answer to these problems is genetic engineering – salmon that grow to seven or eight times normal size at a more rapid rate. All the problems of disease, escapes and pollution would be magnified. A fanciful way around the disease and pollution problems are giant robotic fish farms that will drift across the Atlantic on the Gulf Stream, full of feed and little fish as they float away from Florida, full of big fish by the time they reach Europe.

Freshwater fish farming suffers the usual problems of intensification – a viral herpes-like disease infecting carp was first found in intensive carp ponds in Israel in 1997 and is now wiping out farmed carp populations in Japan and Holland.

There are alternatives to fish that provide comparable nutrients, including seaweed for iodine and hemp, flax seeds and oils for essential fatty acids. However, the sea is a hugely productive resource that could provide us with an endless supply of food if only we were to manage it in a sustainable manner.

• The Marine Stewardship Council scheme guarantees that fish are produced in a sustainable fashion – Thames herring and New Zealand hoki for example.

• The Soil Association certifies the St. Helena fishery in the South Atlantic. It is unpolluted, operated by local fishermen and does not deplete fish stocks.

Marine Stewardship Council
www.msc.org
Seafood Watch
www.mbayaq.org/cr/seafoodwatch.asp
Sea Shepherd Conservation Society
www.seashepherd.com

ANIMAL WELFARE

lives at stake

Most people love animals, but when it comes to eating them, people have ways of resolving the inner conflict between kind feelings for them and an appetite for their flesh, milk or eggs. Animal husbandry, the breeding and rearing of stock animals, has a tradition as long as arable agriculture. Issues of welfare and cruelty have only become a popular concern in the past few decades.

Before the introduction of antibiotics and other disease-suppressing drugs into agriculture, intensification just wasn't possible. If a farmer squeezed too much milk out of a cow, packed too many pigs in a shed or too many chickens in a cage, the animals would die of disease. Farmers knew the limits and those limits corresponded with a reasonable existence for the animals.

The economic advantages of intensification are considerable: reduced housing costs as more animals fit into a smaller space, reduced expenditure on labor and, because the animals don't use up energy walking around, better conversion of feed into meat. The impact on animal behavior is inevitable – they attack each other in the hateful states that intensive habitation induces. To prevent this, chickens are debeaked, piglets have their tails cut off, turkeys have their toes clipped and cattle have their horns removed. Dairy cattle are bred to produce so much milk that their bones crumble after a year or two. Bacterial infection is common, as are metabolic disorders arising from a diet of unnaturally concentrated feeds.

As slaughterhouses become larger and able to process more animals per hour, issues of animal welfare in transport arise. Animals have longer distances to travel to their ultimate fate. 80,000 pigs die in the US every year in transport. Once at the abattoir, pigs that are not successfully stunned are boiled alive in scalding-tanks. Cattle that are improperly stunned bleed to death as their insides fall to the floor.

People suffer, too. Slaughterhouse workers have high accident rates, low pay and psychological disorders.

Consumers are generally disgusted by the idea of cruelty to animals, but many are reluctant to pay the cost for meat produced to higher welfare standards. Periodic exposés lead only to a temporary drop in meat consumption. However, revulsion at farm animal cruelty is a major factor in the growth of vegetarianism. Organic meat does provide an alternative.

Farmers don't voluntarily engage in cruel practice, though they become hardened to suffering after repeated exposure. Faced with the choice between bankruptcy or cruelty to animals, few choose losing their farm. As long as their customers buy only what is cheapest, they will only produce what they can sell profitably.

The EU has introduced welfare standards that improve the worst aspects of animal rearing, including the ending of caged battery chickens by 2012. But the US is going in the opposite direction. Many states have amended their laws to specifically exclude farm animals from anti-cruelty legislation. Consumer concern, however, can and does motivate fast-food companies to act. McDonald's, under pressure from PETA (People for Ethical Treatment of Animals) now buys eggs from suppliers who use larger cages and reject debeaking. They have also told suppliers that by 2005 their pork should be reared without hormones or antibiotics. This will force less cruel and more extensive practices on farmers and lead to improved animal health.

The availability of healthier meat may also help to retard the growth of our own health problems that arise from fatty, diseased, drugged and hormone-implanted meat. Animals' suffering is, ironically, our suffering.

The Food Revolution; John Robbins
Conari Press 2001; ISBN: 1-573-2470-2-2

Batteries Not Included: A Soil Association Report
supported by Compassion in World Farming
ISBN 0-9052009-6-9; www.soilassociation.org

www.cok.net; www.vivausa.org
www.farmsanctuary.org; www.peta.org

FUNCTIONAL FOOD

pharming the food supply

Functional foods burst onto the market in March 2000 with mass media advertising and impressive heath claims. Novartis, a leading pharmaceutical company, launched the "Aviva" range stating: "Substantial benefits in heart, digestive and bone health can all be achieved by an appropriate choice of diet. Eating a balanced diet and taking regular exercise greatly

Functional foods compensate for the junk food diet, lack of exercise and stress of modern life

assist our health and the likelihood of well being in later years. However, the pace and demands of modern living can compromise the feasibility of an optimal lifestyle, reducing

the positive contribution that diet and exercise can make."

In a nutshell, functional foods compensate for the junk food diet, lack of exercise and stress of modern life. In most cases they include healthy ingredients with proven health benefits, but they are usually mixed with the very same foods that cause ill health.

Functional food developed from the involvement of the pharmaceutical industry in food production. Medicine represents one part of their income; food processing another. Out of this melding of food and medicine, functional foods were created to build on the concept of fortified food. A food that has been refined needs to have back some of the nutrients that went missing in the process, or deficiency diseases are a risk. Adding calcium and B vitamins to white bread is a common example. We now know that, as well as vitamins and minerals, processing also discards other important nutrients such as fructo-oligosaccharides, anthyocyanins, betacarotene and phenolic compounds. By adding back a few well-known nutrients, the manufacturer publicizes its set of additives while ignoring the nutrients that are required in a balanced diet.

Diet and nutrition are replacing a reliance on drugs and surgery as the foundation of a healthy life for many people. The trend towards healthy eating is the basis of the organic and natural products industry. Meanwhile, the pharmaceutical industry has thrived by selling drugs to alleviate the symptoms of disease, much of which is caused by poor diet. They've lobbied vigorously to suppress competition from natural products such as herbs and nutritional supplements. With functional food they hope to hitch a ride on the trend towards healthy diet and preventive medicine.

The basic premise of functional food is always the same. Take a poor-quality food, add a few "magic bullets" and sell it as a cure for chronic health problems. The benefits are questionable. Aviva, for example, had three categories of product: Heart Benefits, Bone Benefits and Digestive Benefits:

- Oat bran and Vitamins C & E are added to their Heart Benefits foods to help reduce cholesterol. Oddly, they also contain 20 per cent hydrogenated fat and 40% sugar, which help increase harmful cholesterol.
- Bone Benefits bars contains magnesium and calcium to help replace bone but again, a high level of sugar and hydrogenated fat undermines overall health.

The benefits of functional food are questionable

- Digestive Benefits bars contain 20% fructo-oligosaccharides (FOS). This is a "prebiotic" that helps friendly "probiotic" intestinal bacteria. However, they also contain 40% white sugar, which is what upsets healthful bacteria levels in the first place.

These products rely on the benefits of one ingredient in isolation and ignore powerful negative co-factors such as sugar and hydrogenated fats.

So, how successful are functional foods?

"Out of 1,100 products launched in the nutraceuticals industry last year, only 42 reached $1 million in sales," revealed David Weinberg of Lerner Health Products back in March 2000. That's less than a 4% survival rate.

The confectionery industry is one of the last hopes for functional food. The June 2002 *Candy Industry* magazine comments: "Confectionery manufacturers can take nutritional ingredients and put them in a convenient form that looks and tastes better than a couple of pills." Sugar, associated with heart, bone and digestive

> Truly functional foods such as yogurt and wholewheat bread have been doing their work for millenia

disease, is now seen as the most effective vehicle for delivering isolated healthy ingredients.

The Aviva range was withdrawn after failing to achieve expected sales in the UK, though it is still available via doctors in the US and UK.

Truly "functional" foods such as yogurt, wholewheat bread and oat porridge have been doing their good work for millennia. Adding a few nutritionally valuable ingredients to a junk food diet is a "band-aid" approach that misses the "aware" consumer and is of little interest to the junk-food lover. For some, the presence of a few vitamins or nutrients might compensate for the guilt felt at eating sugary snacks instead of a proper meal.

• Genetic engineering offers the promise of being able to create new functional foods by inserting desirable nutritional characteristics into foods. But can the market for such products, judging by the market problems of existing functional foods, ever repay the development cost?

• For most of us, the answer to our nutritional problems stares us in the face: eat good, natural food.

The Functional Foods Revolution
Michael Heasman, Julian Mellentin
Earthscan 2001
ISBN 1-8538368-7-7

ANTIBIOTICS

the impact on human health

The introduction of penicillin in 1935 heralded a new era in medicine: the development of antibiotics. Diseases which had formerly been incurable could be treated effectively with these new "wonder drugs." Many millions of lives were to be saved. Over time, however, resistance to antibiotics emerged and more and more antibiotics ceased to be effective. Perhaps this was inevitable, but the development of resistance has been accelerated by a number of factors:

- Hospital use of antibiotics to cut cleaning and labor costs in place of expensive sterilization and hygiene methods.
- Unnecessary prescriptions by doctors, often for viral conditions for which they are ineffective, such as the common cold.
- Routine addition of antibiotics to animal feeds as growth promoters.

By killing off an animal's normal digestive flora, antibiotics allow more of the animal's food intake to be converted into flesh. The natural resistance to disease is lost; the antibiotics replace the natural immune function.

More than 70% of all antibiotics used worldwide are used in agriculture. Many of these are identical or very similar to those used in human medicine. When bacteria develop resistance to

Resistance to antibiotics has emerged, with more and more antibiotics becoming ineffective

an antibiotic they can transmit this resistance to other bacteria, rendering medical uses no longer viable.

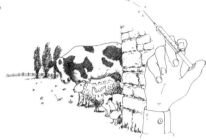

proponents' claims of precision, the inserted genes are unstable. If a GM product is fed to an animal the resistant DNA can be transferred to bacteria in the gut, rendering antibiotics used as medicine useless. Antibiotic-resistant genetic materials now have been abandoned in genetic engineering, but it is still the base of "first generation" genetically engineered animal feed crops on the market.

Staphylococcus aureus (MRSA), a common hospital infection, used to be treated by the "last resort" antibiotic vancomycin until a new variant emerged. The excessive use of avoparcin, a vancomycin-like antibiotic used in agriculture, is probably the cause. Avoparcin was banned in 1997, but by then the resistance

If a GM product is fed to an animal, resistant DNA can render antibiotics used as medicine useless

had been transferred. In Japan some hospitals have been closed and sealed shut in an attempt to contain the resistant bacteria.

Genetic engineering uses antibiotic resistant genes – this presents a further risk. Despite its

Most antibiotics evolved in soil where their function is to help maintain the balance of life in the "soil food web." Antibiotic residues in manure and in slurry runoff from intensive feedlots encourage the development of antibiotic resistant bacteria in soil and in the water supply, further increasing the risk of transferred resistance. Any antibiotic residues that find their way into the food chain upset the natural balance of our intestinal flora and the "digestive food web."

There are a number of regularly consumed foods that are produced with the use of antibiotics. They include:

Chicken – battery chickens for meat are fed growth-promoting antibiotics throughout their lives. Free-range chickens are antibiotic-free.

Turkey – ionophores, a group of drugs known to have neurotoxic effects on animals at low levels, are fed daily to prevent parasite infection. One in four turkeys from a flock in East Anglia didn't make it to the vital Christmas 2001 date because of poisoning from ionophores.

Eggs – though laying hens are not fed antibiotics as growth promoters, they are fed antibiotics to control parasitic diseases that are common in intensive egg-production systems. Residues have been found in eggs.

Beef – feedlot beef cattle, reared on grain, are regularly fed growth-promoting antibiotics. Grass fed cattle are not.

Pork – pig rearing depends heavily on antibiotics. Piglets are weaned prematurely and develop pneumonia easily, requiring treatment with antibiotics. Up to ten different antibiotics are used in pork production, for disease prevention and growth promotion.

Milk – when a milking cow goes dry a few months before giving birth to a calf, a tube of antibiotics is inserted into her udder to prevent bacterial infections. These antibiotics infuse the calf's first milk intake.

Fish – antibiotics in fish farming are commonplace and spread into the environment, affecting wild fish and shellfish.

The factory chicken industry is already walking a tightrope, alternating drugs to an agreed

The factory chicken industry is already walking a tightrope

rotation, hoping to extend the effectiveness of antibiotics. Nonetheless, there have been failures. One large chicken factory has been closed down and the entire building disinfected in order to eliminate resistant strains of disease.

Antibiotics are never routinely used on any animals under organic farming systems. When an organically reared animal is ill, antibiotics may be used as a last resort. If this happens, the animal cannot be sold as organic meat, nor its milk or eggs be sold as "organic" until after a withdrawal period.

In Sweden and Denmark, with government funding assistance, farming standards have changed to avoid the need for antibiotics. Other countries need to make changes, too. It is little help imposing quality standards on domestic producers without controls on imports, as they merely import the resistance problem.

The 1970s saw the last big breakthrough in antibiotic development. A new antibiotic is being trialed – Ziracin – with high hopes for its ability to control hospital "superbugs." Yet even as Ziracin is being tested, an almost identical drug, Avilamycin, is being introduced as a growth

> In Sweden and Denmark, farming standards have changed to avoid the need for antibiotics

promoter to replace four antibiotics that have been banned in chicken production. The risk of further resistance developing is high.

With no new antibiotics in the pipeline, drug companies need to increase sales of existing ones. Advertising in farming magazines encourages excessive antibiotic use, helping to ensure that the consumer gets cheap chicken in the short run but greater risk of dangerous hospital infections in the long run.

In the Northeast US in April 2002 there was an outbreak of *Salmonella* Newport contracted from contaminated hamburger beef. Medical authorities in five states attempted to treat it with nine different antibiotics, all of which had been used against *Salmonella* before. None of them worked. *Salmonella* Newport is becoming increasingly common in beef cattle as it resists all farm antibiotics. Proposals include cleaner production practices or compulsory irradiation of all hamburger meat with Cobalt–60. The real solutions, of course, lie elsewhere.

Superbug
Geoffrey Cannon
Virgin Books 1996
ISBN 0-8636993-4-0

Killer Superbugs.
The Story of Drug-Resistant Diseases
Nancy Day
Enslow Publishers 2000
ISBN 0-7660158-8-2

ADDITIVES

hidden and blatant

"Added value" is the term that processors use to describe the profit from the transformation of natural food stuffs into a ready-to-eat form. Time is money, so the value of processing represents the saving of the customer's time. Nutritional value, however, can often be lost.

The adulteration of food has a long and inglorious history. Medieval bakers were marched in shackles through the streets, pelted with rotten fruit and abuse, for the addition of finely ground chalk and sawdust to add whiteness and weight to bread. Water was added to milk or wine, pig's blood gave color to stale fish. Brick dust was added to cocoa, red lead gave the deep orange color to Gloucester cheeses, used tea leaves were dyed with black lead.

A modern processor can make a profit in two ways: by improving ingredients in a way that is difficult for a cook at home, or by diluting the character of the food – by adding ingredients that cost less than the food itself. The cheapest are air and water, the processor's favorites. But they come with problems:

* loss of flavor
* loss of color
* loss of texture
* poor appearance
* risk of microbial attack and oxidation

So, artificial flavorings, colorings, bulking agents and preservatives are added to mask the loss

Artificial flavorings, colorings and preservatives mask quality loss

of quality. The Federal Food and Drugs Acts in 1906 sought to prevent "the manufacture, sale, or transportation of adulterated or misbranded or poisonous or deleterious foods, drugs, medicines and liquors." Much of the ensuing debate about food quality and purity has revolved around the definition of its terminology. Subsequent legislation includes the "Delaney Clause," an amendment that bans the approval for use in food of any additive which is shown to cause cancer in humans or animals. However, there are already additives in use that are "prior sanctioned" or "GRAS" (Generally Recognized As Safe) which are permitted on the basis that they have been used for some time with no known harmful effects. Until these additives are tested in isolation it is impossible to be sure that they are safe. As evidence has

If an additive causes allergic reactions such as asthma, there is no legislative barrier to its use

emerged of risk, many additives on the GRAS list have been removed. How many more could withstand serious scrutiny?

In addition, scientists can argue about whether a substance is carcinogenic or not, while its potential as a mutagen or teratogen or allergen

may be overlooked. The research, which enables the FDA to determine which additives may be used, is funded by the manufacturers of the additives, not by independent laboratories or by the FDA itself. There is, therefore potential for "wishful thinking" in the construction of studies and the methodology of trials. If an additive causes allergic reactions such as asthma, or digestive reactions such as irritable bowel syndrome or Crohn's Disease there is no legislative barrier to its use in food.

Why the concern?

Additives are a worry because, among other things, they affect learning ability in children cause hyperactivity and can be hormone disruptors, carcinogens and mutagens.

Legislation on food labeling might appear to be the answer. However, it enables processors to avoid the issue because there are some additives that don't have to be listed on product labels. For example ingredients such as "broth," "natural flavor" or "spices" may contain other ingredients and these do not have to listed on the label, so even the most careful reading of an ingredients list will not inform the consumer of what additives may be present. This provides a hiding place where a manufacturer can conceal the existence of an ingredient that they fear may deter a customer from purchasing the product.

Reading the label

"Natural" flavorings are not natural. They have the same chemical formula as the ingredient found in nature, but are made from petrochemicals. They are more durable than the natural flavors to which they are "identical" and cannot be detected by analysis. "Natural flavor" is derived from a natural source.

"Flavoring" can indicate the presence of monosodium glutamate or hydrolyzed vegetable protein (see chapter "Tastes Familiar"). Artificial flavors compensate for the lack of taste in poor-quality products, particularly factory-farmed meat. Cured smoked bacon is expensive to produce; smoke flavoring and artificial coloring are cheaper. Tasteless broiler chicken is tumbled in a liquid solution that contains hydrolyzed beef or pork extracts to infuse it with flavor and increase its weight by up to 30%. The addition of water need not be declared unless it exceeds statutory permitted levels (10% of the weight of the meat).

Colorings are a particularly sensitive subject. Tartrazine, a popular yellow color, causes hyperactive behavior and violence in children.

Hydrogenated fat, with its plastic-like hardness, adds structure and texture to industrially produced biscuits and bread. More air and water can then be added without the end product collapsing or crumbling.

Preservatives are particularly important when water has been added to a product. Many foods

A popular yellow coloring causes violence in children

have a natural stability which helps them to resist deterioration and microbial attack. However, if a product has been injected with water this resistance is lost and preservatives are needed to protect it from the development of pathogens. Preservatives, like antibiotics, randomly kill bacteria and so also affect the digestive flora of the gut (see chapter "The Digestive System").

Not all foods have to declare all their ingredients. Wine and beer contain a wide variety of adulterants, colorings, flavors, preservatives and processing aids that are excluded from labeling requirements. Confectionery and chocolate products sold loose also escape labeling law. Food sold in restaurants and fast food outlets does not come with an ingredient listing. Genetically engineered food, with added DNA, is not labeled as such.

Organic food regulations only allow a handful of permitted food additives and those are all of natural origin, such as soy lecithin or citric acid. Organic labels must also declare all ingredients, regardless of percentage content – so no hidden additives.

A consumer cannot make an informed choice about food unless the information is available

Organic food regulations only allow a handful of permitted food additives of natural origin

on packaging. This may present some difficulties to packaging designers but how else are we to trust our food?

• "Golden Fields" white bread sold in New York contains "20% fiber from natural forest sources"; they've put the sawdust back in bread. Calcium carbonate (chalk) is added to white bread to boost its calcium content. Medieval bakers would be amused to discover that their adulterants are now marketed as healthy additives.

• A popular 19th Century story told of the customer who asked for a discount on sausages as he'd been a loyal customer for seven years. "Seven years!" exclaimed the butcher, "and you're still alive?"

Food Additives (2004 Revised Edition)
Christine H. Farlow
Kiss for Health Publications 2004
ISBN 0-9635635-4-6

A Consumer's Dictionary of Food Additives
Ruth Winter
Three Rivers Press 1999
ISBN 0-6098036-6-2

WHOLEGRAINS

the perfect food

Every great civilization of history has been founded on whole cereal grains. Civilizations evolved when a farmer managed to produce enough wholegrains to feed himself, his family and have a surplus to share with his community. In turn, the people who asserted control over the food supply – warriors, priests and princes – prospered. Nutritionally, wholegrains provided such a sound dietary foundation that the vagaries of the rest of the diet did not undermine overall health.

A recommended modern diet can be represented by the Harvard School of Public Health "Healthy Eating Food Pyramid," with wholegrain cereal foods as the basis of a healthy diet. This version of the Food Pyramid has been shown to deliver 40% reductions in heart disease risk and 20% reductions in chronic disease risk compared to the USDA Food Pyramid, which doesn't differentiate wholegrains from low fiber foods such as white bread, white rice, pasta and potatoes. The arguments for such a recommendation are strong.

Wholegrains protect against cancer, (particularly stomach and colon cancer), and reduce the risk of coronary heart disease, diabetes and hypertension – all this because of their high content of dietary fiber, starch, oligosaccharides, trace minerals, vitamins, antioxidants and phytoestrogens.

Wholegrains include wheat, rice, maize (corn), oats, rye, barley, sorghum and millet. Whole wheat and brown rice each represent 31% of the world's grain production. However, 21% is milled white rice. The other 10% – rice bran and germ – goes for animal feed. Each year nearly 440 billion pounds of highly nutritious rice bran and germ and a further 220 billion pounds of wheat germ and bran are refined out of the human food chain. This represents 660 billion pounds per annum of nutritious food for each of the 1 billion people on the planet who go to bed hungry.

A whole cereal grain contains three main parts: the endosperm, germ and bran. Endosperm is mostly carbohydrate, with up to 10% protein. The germ is rich in nutrients including vitamins, minerals and oils. The bran is the outer casing and is also known as "dietary fiber."

Until recent times, most grains were ground on millstones. To remove some of the bran and germ it was "bolted" – shaken through a coarse material – to give fine whiteish flour. This was an expensive process, so white bread was a luxury reserved for the wealthy.

The first roller mills appeared in the 1880s. Now the bran and the germ could be removed separately to leave white flour. White bread became available to the masses. The nutritious germ and bran were sold for animal feed or to early health-food suppliers.

When industrial rice mills were introduced into Asia, and white rice became easily available, outbreaks of beri-beri were noted. This is a Vitamin B1-deficiency disease that leads to numbness, confusion and mental instability. Experiments in the Kuala Lumpur Lunatic Asylum in Malaya in 1907 published in *The Lancet* showed that substituting brown rice for white cured mental illness. As a reaction, "parboiled" rice is now eaten widely where rice is a staple. In this process, wholegrain "paddy" rice is steeped in hot water long enough for the B vitamins in the rice bran to soak into the grain and so help prevent beri-beri.

In the West, the main result of eating more white bread was constipation and a burgeoning market for laxatives. But millers were happy because white flour meant fewer pest problems – insects cannot survive or reproduce on a diet of white flour. By the 1940s, however, it was clear that white bread was nutritionally inadequate and "fortification,"

> In the West, the main result of eating more white bread was constipation and a burgeoning market for laxatives

the adding back of missing nutrients, became mandatory for white flour.

What are the benefits of Wholegrains?

All grains contain a balance of carbohydrate and protein that corresponds closely to the balance needed in our diet. But wholegrains have more.

Fermentable Carbohydrates

Wholegrains contain high levels of "fermentable carbohydrate," including dietary fiber and oligosaccharides. These keep the contents of the intestine moving and gently scour away any accumulations of fiber-free sticky foods such as cheese, beef or white flour. This hurries food through the digestive system, ensuring that toxins are excreted before they can be reabsorbed. These carbohydrates aren't digested in the small intestine but are fermented in the colon by intestinal flora to produce short chain fatty acids. The best known of these is butyrate, important in maintaining the health of the cells in the colon, decreasing the risk of cancer.

Blood Sugar Levels

The dietary fiber of wholegrains also slows the rate of digestion and absorption of carbohydrates.

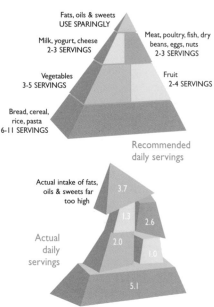

Recommended daily servings

Actual daily servings

This helps moderate blood sugar levels, reducing the risk of obesity and diabetes.

Prebiotics

These are the non-digestible carbohydrates, or "fructo-oligosaccharides" (FOS), that nourish the "friendly" intestinal flora.

Wholegrains are rich in vitamins, trace minerals and a variety of phytonutrients that protect against cancer and ageing. They are an excellent source of vitamin E and selenium.

What's more, wholegrains, properly prepared, taste delicious and their bulk discourages

> Wholegrains are the most economic use of the Earth's food-producing resources and are a sustainable way of maintaining health

overeating because they give a sense of fullness. They are the most economic use of the Earth's food-producing resources and represent a sustainable way of maintaining health.

Hope's Edge: The Next Diet for a Small Planet
Frances Moore Lappé, Anna Lappé
Jeremy P. Tarcher 2002
ISBN 1-5854214-9-9

NUTRITION AND FOOD QUALITY

getting what we need

What makes food good for you? Is it just the primary nutrients such as vitamins, minerals, carbohydrates, fat and protein content? The discovery of vitamin and mineral deficiency-related diseases was a major breakthrough in nutrition studies and led to the fortification of refined foods such as white bread and breakfast cereals. Or is there more to food than A, B and C?

Since 1940, McCance and Widdowson's *Composition of Foods* has analyzed and recorded the nutritional content of a wide variety of foods. In that time key minerals in food have decreased by 40%, reflecting the decline in mineral content of soil since the widespread use of agrichemicals began. Plants grown with agrichemicals do not develop the same healthy defenses as plants grown organically because pesticides and artificial fertilizers replace many of the normal functions of the plant. A healthy plant has its own immune system and secretes substances that help it deal with the stress of disease and insect attack. These are the micronutrients, many of which – flavonoids and anthocyanins for example – are antioxidants. They have only recently been recognized as important in neutralizing the "free radicals" in food that induce cancer and other diseases. Eating these healthy plants

Key minerals in food have decreased by 40% since 1940

can make an important contribution to the health of an animal or human being. Flavonoids help regulate our hormones and cell growth. Anthocyanins help eye function and the nervous system. Terpenes such as carotenoids prevent breast and prostate cancers. Sulfur-containing glucosinolates and allicins prevent cancer, help heavy metal removal and protect the heart. The *Composition of Foods* doesn't have measurements of these micro-nutrients dating back 50 years. It is, however, now known that when plants get high levels of artificial nitrogen fertilizer and are sprayed with pesticides and

Organic food contains higher levels of Vitamin C, iron, magnesium and phosphorous

fungicides they produce much lower levels, not just of the main vitamins and minerals, but of these key nutritive elements as well. The "Worthington Report" in 2001 established that organic food contained significantly higher levels of Vitamin C, iron, magnesium and phosphorous and significantly fewer nitrates than conventional crops.

Thus, the question as to whether organic carrots have higher levels of vitamin A or not is of interest because it indicates whether other important nutrients are also present. We are looking at the immune system of the carrot.

What about the essential vitality of food? We instinctively know that the healthier food is, the more likely it is to do us good. Given the choice between a sick, crippled chicken with missing feathers or a fit, healthy one with glossy plumage, we'd rather eat the healthy bird that exhibits all the signs of natural vitality. It takes little imagination to conclude that if these plants and animals thrive on an organic system, the same must be true for human beings too.

Because of the economic importance of livestock, many advances in nutritional understanding come from research into animal health rather than human health. This may sound strange, but a sick animal is a financial loss to a farmer whereas a sick human, paradoxically, represents income opportunities for the medical industry. Animal feeds are carefully mixed to ensure that deficiencies are minimized. Feeding trials have shown that animals decline in health over generations if fed on foods grown with fertilizers and pesticides. Reproductive and sperm motility problems occur. Some breeders choose organically grown feed to maintain desirable genetic traits in their animals. For example, swan breeders buy aquatic weed seeds purchased from organic rice growers to ensure that ornamental characteristics are passed on. Racing stables often use organic oats.

It's easy when you're feeding an animal – it has no freedom of choice. We can't, however, coerce people to eat well. So, it is essential that we be persuaded to eat wholesome food, rather than junk food.

• In 1936, The American Senate gave the following warning: "The alarming fact is that foods (fruits, vegetables and grains) now being raised on millions of acres of land that no longer contain enough of certain minerals are starving us – no matter how much of them we eat. No man of today can eat enough fruits and vegetables to supply his system with the minerals he requires for perfect health because his stomach isn't big enough to hold them." The 1930s saw the Dust Bowl and the erosion of large parts of America's soil as the fertility of the prairies was finally used up. Agrichemical use kept the exhausted land in production but the missing minerals were never replaced, except on organic farms.

• In August 2000, King's College in London released the results of a research study: between 10% and 30% of adolescent girls have mild iron deficiency, and those girls who were iron deficient had a significantly lower I.Q.

The Encyclopedia of Natural Medicine
Michael Murray, Joseph Pizzorno
Prima Lifestyles
ISBN 0-7615115-7-1

BRAIN FOOD

think about it

"Jeeves is incredible in the brain-power department. He puts it down to the fact that he eats almost nothing but fish."
Bertie Wooster, P.G. Wodehouse

The healthy brain relies on a constant supply of essential nutrients – all of which come from the food we eat. Any interference, either in the

Half of the brain's DHA is formed while in the womb

growing or processing of food, that affects the nutritional make-up directly affects our body's ability to function properly. A few examples will show how important a balanced diet is to our general health.

Essential Fatty Acids

Oily fish such as herring, mackerel, sardines, salmon and tuna are rich sources of substances known as Essential Fatty Acids (EFAs) essential for effective food metabolism and for the regulation of cell growth and regeneration. Docosahexaenoic acid (DHA), for example builds brain structure. 50% of the brain's DHA is formed while in the womb and the remainder in the first year of the baby's life.

So, Jeeves' legendary brain power owed as much to his mother's diet as it did to his own food choices. DHA is transmitted through the placenta and mother's milk, so the prenatal diet is vital. This period of brain growth is the baby's only chance to develop its full potential; it can't make up the deficit later in life. But eating fish later in life does help to maintain the brain.

EFAs are crucial for brain function, good vision memory and learning. Research has shown that fish oil supplements help children with dyslexia hyperactivity and even autism. In older people senile dementia and schizophrenia are linked to diets low in DHA.

Taking fish oil as a supplement is a quick fix rather than a solution for DHA deficiency, though. Fish oil comes from the same sources that produce feed for intensive poultry, pig and salmon farms. It also comes with all the risks of pollutants that accumulate in fish, such as dioxins and PCBs.

Vegetarian parents need not worry, however. Non-fish eaters can still enjoy high DHA levels because healthy cells manufacture DHA from the "omega-3" essential fatty acids found in vegetables. This function, however, is impaired by hydrogenated fat, frying oil, rancid oil, alcohol and excess cholesterol from animal products. It also is reduced by ageing, diabetes, low blood sugar and infections.

Omega-3 EFAs can be found in flax, hemp and pumpkin seeds, or their oils. Tofu, tempeh and dark green vegetables such as kale and parsley, as well as wheat grass and spirulina are also good sources. All chlorophyll cells in plants contain omega-3 so cows that graze mainly on grass have omega-3 in their meat and milk. Intensively reared cattle have high levels of saturated fat and little omega-3.

Iodine

The thyroid gland relies on the mineral iodine to produce its hormone, thyroxine, used to control metabolic rates, energy levels and brain development. The mental condition

Iodine must be consumed regularly to maintain healthy levels

"cretinism" was first diagnosed among Swiss children in mountain areas with no iodine content in the soil. In the 1930s, 40% of the people in Michigan had goiter, a symptom of iodine deficiency. Most of the world's iodine-deficient areas do not require the compulsory iodization of salt (although Vietnam and India are beginning to iodize). Iodine readily washes out of soil so its best dietary source is from sea vegetables and fish – kelp tablets and sushi rolls for examples. And because iodine is not stored in the body, it must be consumed regularly to maintain healthy levels.

Antioxidants

"Free radicals" – reactive oxidant particles – damage the fatty brain-cell membranes making them susceptible to disease. Antioxidants help minimize free radical damage. Vitamins C and E, coenzyme Q10, betacarotene (found in dark-colored fruits and vegetables including carrots and parsley) and flavonoids (including tea) all act as antioxidants. Vitamin E is found in whole grains but not in refined flour products.

Blood sugar and oxygen

The levels of iron, glucose and oxygen in your blood make a big difference to brain function. Iron is a major component of hemoglobin

> A diet rich in whole grains and vegetables will provide nutrition for the brain

in red blood cells, needed to carry oxygen around the body. High iron levels ensure high oxygen levels which, as long as there is enough glucose available for the process of metabolism, ensures that the brain can function at maximum capability. Taking a walk after a meal helps oxygenate the brain.

Amino acids

The neurotransmitters in the brain, that carry messages from one neuron cell to the next, are made from proteins, themselves made up of amino acids. Of the 20 naturally occurring amino acids, some are created in the body, others we have to obtain from the food we eat. These are called "essential" amino acids and can be gained from a balanced diet.

Of course, the brain responds to factors other than diet. Lead, in the air and in drinking water should be avoided, as should stress and noise. Physical and mental exercise, relaxation and adequate sleep all help. A diet rich in whole grains and vegetables will provide nutrition for the brain, with oily fish providing a back-up supply when needed.

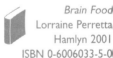

Brain Food
Lorraine Perretta
Hamlyn 2001
ISBN 0-6006033-5-0

HYDROGENATION OF FAT

butter wouldn't melt

Fats, perhaps because of the association with obesity, are sometimes seen as "bad" food in the diet, to be avoided whenever possible. However, essential fatty acids (EFAs) are a vital part of a healthy diet and underpin the healthy functioning of the nervous system, not least fetal brain development. Yet we see the strange paradox in the USA where daily consumption of essential fatty acids is two to three times the required level, and still people suffer from heart disease, cancer and skin disease – diseases that are directly associated with EFA deficiencies. Why is this? Let's consider hydrogenated fats.

What is Hydrogenation?

Hydrogenated fat is usually made with soy or cottonseed oil that has been refined in a process that involves crushing the seeds in a hexane solvent. Like its related chemicals (methane, propane, octane and heptane), hexane is highly inflammable, even explosive, but it also separates the oil from the rest of the seed and is then recovered by evaporation, leaving pure and, it is hoped, solvent-free vegetable oil.

The resulting vegetable oil is mixed with nickel particles and heated to 200°C. The mixture is then held at this temperature for up to six hours while hydrogen gas is pumped through at high pressure. The bonds within the oil molecules are weakened to breaking point, making them vulnerable to invasion by atoms that wouldn't

Essential fatty acids underpin a healthy nervous system

normally be able to penetrate. The hydrogen atoms lodge in the oil molecules and form "trans fats," new and complex substances that don't exist in nature. Once cooled, this fat is very hard and can be stored as plastic-like beads for use in the manufacture of many common foods including:

- Margarine – using hydrogenated fat enables a higher level of polyunsaturates, but only at the cost of having a high level of trans fats.
- Bread – hydrogenated fat enables the loaf to have a higher water and air content, giving the appearance of greater bulk.
- Chips and snacks – deep fried foods have a drier, less oily texture as the trans fats do not melt at room temperatures.
- Biscuits and crackers – hydrogenated fat gives a crisper, less oily feel.

Professor Walter Willett at Harvard University conducted a study of 67,000 nurses who kept dietary records for 12 years. The results, published in 1993 in the

> Hydrogenated fat consumption is directly related to increased rates of hearth diseases and cancer

New England Journal of Medicine, were conclusive: hydrogenated fat consumption is directly related to increased rates of heart disease, cancer, obesity and skin disease. The authors wrote: "Our findings must add to the concern that the practice of partially hydrogenating vegetable oils may have reduced the anticipated benefits of substituting these oils for highly saturated fats, and instead contributed to the occurrence of coronary heart disease."

Organic food regulations worldwide prohibit the use of hydrogenated fat. Meanwhile, hydrogenated fats still make up 30% of the average person's fat intake, with the highest proportion among the lowest income groups, who consume less olive oil or butter and more margarine.

Why is Hydrogenation harmful?

Trans fats are so hard that you can hold them in your hand all day and they won't melt. When we eat fats they are absorbed into the system by fat receptors. But when these receptors receive hydrogenated fats they aren't quite sure what to do with them and they hold on to them. Imagine a line at a ticket window where the person at the front can't decide what ticket to buy. People further back will drift away hoping to get through elsewhere. The same happens with hydrogenated fats: they clog up the fat receptors and the EFAs can't get through and end up being lost. So a person whose diet includes plenty of EFAs can still suffer from EFA deficiency. One way around this is to consume directly the oils that EFAs are converted to – hemp oil, evening primrose oil, flax oil and fish oils, for example. Better still, avoid hydrogenated fat in the first place.

Health implications

It was Willett's report that first brought hydrogenated trans fats under scrutiny. Recent studies have further confirmed trans fats as a major dietary health hazard. When McDonald's switched from using beef tallow to hydrogenated fat in 1990, the trans fat content of their french fries rose from 5% of overall fat to 43%. The Community Nutrition Institute (CNI) in Washington, D.C. attacked McDonald's for this decision, stating that incidents of heart disease, obesity and diabetes would rise as a result. Rodney Leonard of the CNI claimed that the "killer fries" would:

• lead to involuntary obesity. Despite the same caloric intake and exercise levels, people who regularly eat hydrogenated fats weigh at least 6 1/2 to 11 pounds more than infrequent users.

• reduce sperm count in males and raise frequency of deformed sperm.
• if eaten by expectant mothers lead to lower weight babies since trans fats interfere in the synthesis of important regulators of the birth process called prostaglandins. Michel Odent, the French natural birth pioneer, links the low consumption of hydrogenated fat in Japan with the comparatively low level of Caesarian and induced deliveries.

In 2004, at the Food and Beverage Conference in London, a senior vice president of McDonald's announced proudly that they had substantially reduced the trans fat content of their foods in

A person whose diet includes plenty of EFAs can still be deficient

Britain, while admitting that they "still had a long way to go" to do the same in the USA.

However, labeling of trans fats on grocery packaging will be compulsory in the US in 2006 – already Oreos have had trans fats removed. In Britain, Mars bars (3 million sold every day) went trans fats-free in 2003 and the 6 million "digestive biscuits" Brits eat every day had trans fats removed in 2004. Other big manufacturers are following suit.

• The other names under which hydrogenated fat appears include, "vegetable margarine," "vegetable fat," "vegetable shortening," "hardened fat" and "vegetable fats and oils."

• "Vegetable oil" is the only description that guarantees no hydrogenation. "Partially

"Partially hydrogenated oil" contains the highest levels of trans fats

hydrogenated oil" is actually the worst, as it contains the highest levels of trans fats. Vanaspati or "vegetable ghee" has the highest level of trans fats of any commonly used shortening and is frequently found in Indian cooking.

Fats That Heal, Fats That Kill
Udo Erasmus
Alive Book 1993
ISBN 0-9204703-8-6

MICROWAVES

soaking up some rays

A pocket full of melted chocolate led to the discovery of microwaves. An engineer working with early magnetrons, the microwave generators that are used in radar, reached into his pocket for a chocolate bar, only to get his fingers covered in goo. By 1947 the first microwave oven, the Raytheon "Radarange," appeared.

The real boost for microwaves came from a combination of the growth of fast food, suburbia and freezer ownership. Food that had home-cooked appeal could be made on assembly lines, frozen and then reheated quickly in fast-food restaurants. Busy mothers could recapture lost time by buying frozen food, and still present the family a choice of different meals, available in minutes. The traditional family dinner was the casualty. Parents and kids no longer got together at least once a day for a meal and a talk. Junior could run in the door, "nuke" some burgers and fries and dash off to meet his friends with barely a word exchanged.

Boiling, roasting, baking and grilling all work by transferring heat from a source into the food. The molecules of the food itself don't change, they just get warmer. Microwaves work differently. Every food molecule has a positive and negative pole, just like a magnet. Microwave energy alternates between positive

The traditional family dinner was the casualty of the microwave

and negative polarity billions of times a second and the same oscillation is induced in the molecules of food, particularly water. This agitation, as the molecules spin back and forth, creates friction that warms up the food. It also deforms the molecular structure of the food. In genetic engineering, microwaves are used to weaken molecular structure to make it easier to insert new genes.

So is it safe to use microwave ovens?

One thing is for sure – if microwaves melt the chocolate bars in your pocket, think about what they would do to parts of your body. By 1971, safety standards to restrict radiation from microwaves had been introduced to protect domestic users and workers in fast-food restaurants from the damaging effects of radiation. Microwave owners are advised to check for loose door hinges and most

> If microwaves melt chocolate, think about what they would do to parts of your body

manufacturers offer specialist services to check that emission levels are safe. Few microwave owners, however, actually call on this service.

But what about the food itself?

When microwaved food comes out of the microwave it is still buzzing with wave energy. So it's a good idea to let it settle down before eating – it can be unexpectedly hot. (Care should always be taken if microwaving a baby's bottle.) Microwaving changes the structure of food and produces radiolytic by-products, new molecules that don't occur in nature. Concern about such changes has led to research and a report in The Lancet in 1989 referred to the conversion of trans amino acids into non-nutritious forms in baby formula. One amino acid, L-proline, was converted into a form that harms the nervous system and kidneys.

A Swiss clinical study found that people who had eaten microwaved food showed a decrease in the blood level of hemoglobin, which carries oxygen to the cells. White blood cell counts also decreased, reducing immune function. When this research was published in 1993 the Swiss electrical products dealers obtained a gagging order on the scientists who did the research. The scientists appealed to the European Court of Human Rights in 1998 and the gag was lifted.

In Russia, where microwaves have been banned since 1976, tests on food quality have found that microwaving formed carcinogens in meat, dairy products, fruit and vegetables and increased the cell-damaging and cancer-causing free radical content of root vegetables. Damage to the "phytonutrients" in food, such as alkaloids, glucosides, galactosides and nitrilosides, was also noted. We are still discovering the nutritional relevance of these "secondary metabolites."

Modern fan-assisted ovens are a better option. They don't emit radiation and they heat food almost as quickly as microwaves by using forced natural convection. At the same time the pleasures of cooking and of gathering for a meal with friends and family are being actively rediscovered, with the "Slow Food" movement at the vanguard (see chapter "Slow Food"). Microwaves do not play a role in this cultural renaissance.

Increased consumer awareness has encouraged restaurant owners to show when foods have been microwaved. As with information about genetic engineering, pesticide content and organic and regional origin, this knowledge empowers the consumer and almost always leads to higher food quality.

VEGETARIANS

eating with conscience

"It is my view that the vegetarian manner of living, by its purely physical effect on the human temperament, would most beneficially influence the lot of mankind."
Albert Einstein 1879-1955

Many people will confess to thinking of vegetarians – let alone vegans – as slightly oddball. But let us consider the situation.

In the US nine million turkeys, chickens, pigs and cows are slaughtered every day. In Great

The arguments for vegetarianism are convincing – morally, economically and environmentally

Britain 3,000 animals are killed for food – every minute. Meanwhile, major world religions such as Judaism, Islam, Christianity, Buddhism and Hinduism include vegetarianism among their core precepts.

Jews and Muslims get around the clear injunction to eschew the consumption of blood by draining the blood from the animal at the slaughterhouse. Buddhists in countries like Thailand employ Muslims to slaughter their meat, thereby absolving themselves of the act of killing.

Why, despite the repeated arguments from religious leaders, philosophers and health experts, do we still eat meat? The arguments for vegetarianism are convincing – morally, economically, environmentally and in terms of health.

Morally, there is the rule "Thou shalt not kill." Most people recoil from killing animals. It is the disconnection between liking animals and having to kill them to eat meat that persuades many people to become vegetarian. Since Pythagoras' time philosophers have linked a vegetarian lifestyle with peace, arguing that, once we are desensitized to killing animals, the killing of fellow humans becomes merely a question of degree rather than an absolute moral restraint. War becomes more likely, peace harder to sustain.

The combined weight of cattle on our planet exceeds that of human beings. To support this, one quarter of the earth's surface is used as livestock pasture. In the US three quarters of all grains and beans produced become animal feed. It takes seven pounds of corn and soybeans to produce one pound of beef, three pounds to produce a pound of chicken. Much of the destruction of the rain forests in Brazil has been to support soybean production for export as animal feed.

95% of food poisoning cases are caused by animal products. The British Medical Association in 1998 announced: "The current state of food safety in the UK is such that all raw meat should be assumed to be contaminated with pathogenic organisms." The intensification of animal production means that animals ingest the feces of fellow animals, increasing the risk of disease. So, in crowded conditions antibiotics are essential ingredients of feed, yet inevitably in such conditions bacteria emerge which are antibiotic-resistant.

In 1983, *E.coli* O157:H7 was first diagnosed as a disease. Nobody is sure why the *E.coli* organism, most often found in ground beef, suddenly mutated into a more virulent, even fatal

Vegetarians have lower mortality from heart disease and cancer

form. (Perhaps because the gene for virulence is located next to the gene for antibiotic resistance.) Two hundred Americans a year now die from *E.coli,* and the second largest cause of kidney failure among American boys is *E.coli* infection. Heart disease and arthritis are linked to a meat-based diet, while bowel cancer is linked to beef consumption. The World Cancer Research Fund has shown that vegetarians have lower overall mortality from, as well as lower risk of, heart disease, obesity and cancers.

According to a 2002 Time/CNN Harris Interactive Survey, 6% of the US population say they never eat meat, rising to 10% in the 25-34-year-old group. The Vegetarian Resource Group estimates that about 1.5% of the US population are vegans, most famously the musician Moby.

Vegans go a step further and avoid all dairy products and eggs. Dairy products depend on the lactation of female livestock following the

A healthy vegan can claim higher absorption of nutrients and a lower intake of saturated fats

birth of young. These calves, lambs and kids are slaughtered (particularly if male and therefore not future milk-producers) as they compete with humans for their mother's milk. Thus the concerns for animal welfare are not fully met by vegetarianism. The use of vast land and economic resources for the production of dairy products and eggs is also an issue, and a healthy vegan can claim higher absorption of nutrients and a lower intake of saturated fats.

Vegetarianism and veganism are growing rapidly now, and choosing a meatless meal,

even for those who don't describe themselves as vegetarian, is a much more common option. Burger King doesn't mention the word "Vegetarian" or "Vegan" in advertising their "BK Veggie" burger – what would have been strange just a few decades ago is now increasingly normal.

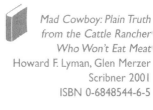

Mad Cowboy: Plain Truth from the Cattle Rancher Who Won't Eat Meat
Howard F. Lyman, Glen Merzer
Scribner 2001
ISBN 0-6848544-6-5

www.vegsource.com

FASTING

take a break

Most of us would be horrified at the thought of going for 40 years of our working life without a vacation, or even a weekend off. Some sacrifices are truly above and beyond the call of duty. Health, happiness and sanity depend on a break from the relentless routine. The brain needs a good night's sleep to recover from a day of thinking. Yet the digestive system works 24 hours a day for a lifetime without getting a chance to rest and recuperate.

The digestive systems of most people in the "rich" world have never been empty from the moment of birth to the moment of death. There's always something in transit, always work to do.

The benefits of fasting have a long history in natural medicine and a far longer one in religion, where the spiritual benefits have an honorable tradition. We chafe at the restrictions and demands that society places upon us and long for freedom to do as we like. But we rarely chafe at the tyranny of the stomach, ever demanding, repeating its call on us to feed it several times a day. How could a complex and sophisticated creation such as a human being have become so abjectly dependent on a regular intake of food?

So, what happens if you don't eat? Quite a lot, and that's why for most generally healthy people it's such a good idea to fast occasionally.

There's no need to go off into the wilderness for 40 days and 40 nights. An 18-hour fast is a simple starter challenge. Eat dinner in the evening. Then don't eat until 2pm the following day. If that is manageable, try a 24-hour fast. Eat an evening meal, then skip breakfast and lunch the next day. Now you're ready for a 36 hour fast – don't eat at all the following day, then "break fast" on the morning of the next day.

Ultimately, the point of fasting is cleansing and rehabilitation. Just as you would drain the oil from a car before adding new oil, so it is beneficial to let the body clear out accumulated wastes from time to time before eating again. It's inner spring cleaning. Fresh air, sunshine and exercise make it more effective.

What happens when you fast?

- The stomach gets a rest, returns to its normal size and rebuilds its hydrochloric acid level.
- The liver continues to regulate blood sugar level but it can also concentrate on getting

> The average Westerner carries five pounds of residues in the colon, mostly from low-fiber foods

rid of unwanted material.
- The pancreas, no longer dealing with unexpected intakes of sugars and no longer producing digestive enzymes, takes a well-earned break.
- The intestines recover their natural tone and the intestinal flora returns to optimal levels, reducing yeasts and fungal organisms.
- Parasites diminish or die.

Most waste accumulates in the colon and it is here that distortion and loss of tone is greatest if we eat too much. The average Westerner carries five pounds of residues in the colon, mostly from low-fiber foods that have not made it through to excretion. Because this waste is usually absorbed back into the bloodstream, getting rid of it leads directly to feeling better, clearer skin, even clearer thoughts. Some people accelerate this cleansing with colonic irrigation – a very personal choice.

If you stop drinking tea or coffee during a fast after a day or two you will begin to experience caffeine withdrawal symptoms that include headaches and deep fatigue. These are the side effects of fasting and getting rid of toxins in the blood. It may be wise to drink small amounts of watery tea or coffee to minimize the impact of withdrawal – unless you intend to break caffeine addiction as a long-term goal.

Once you have fasted for short periods you will know how far you want to go. For a longer fast it may be best to begin with a "semi-fast." Rather than just water, have vegetable juices a few times a day. The seven-day brown rice diet

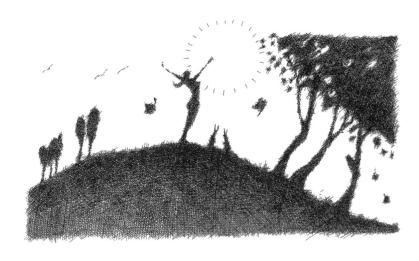

of macrobiotics is another effective way; you learn to enjoy simple food and learn to chew.

With practice, fasting becomes much easier. Fasting with others reduces the sense of isolation and offers mutual support. There is a feeling of freedom and self-reliance that successfully completing a planned fast brings. Once you've done it you'll be hooked.

• If you have weak kidneys, diabetes or any health problem that fasting might exacerbate, then seek professional advice before embarking on a fast.

Fasting-And Eating-For Health: A Medical Doctor's Program for Conquering Disease
Joel Fuhrman
St. Martin's Press 1998
ISBN 0-3121871-9-X

FOREIGN CLIMES

positive approaches to agriculture

Different countries take different approaches to food and farming. Public-private partnerships in some countries have brought enormous benefits.

When Austria first applied for membership in the EU in the early 1990s, the "first-come, first-served" principle of the Common Agricultural Policy (CAP) meant that Austrian farmers wouldn't get the same helpings from the gravy train as those of original member countries such

> Government policy ensured that both Austria's environment and farmers have done well

as Germany, France and Italy. So the Austrian government decided to go for the niche market of organics and by the time Austria was a full member of the EU 9% of its farmland was organic. It produced so much organic corn and potatoes that it became a net exporter of corn for animal feed, corn syrup sweeteners, corn starch, corn grits for breakfast cereals and dried potato products. Foresight and government policy ensured that both Austria's sensitive environment and anxious farmers have done well out of EU entry.

In 1990 in Schleswig-Holstein, the north German state that includes Hamburg and Kiel, the state government encouraged farmers to go organic. Because much of its land is at or below sea-level, the build-up of pesticides and other agricultural pollutants had become insupportable. But farmers expressed concern. They could sell organic vegetables and flax seeds, but what about the organic flax fibers? So the University of Kiel set up a commercial joint venture – Holstein Flachs – to develop organic linen fabrics for clothing and furnishing.

ORGANIC LAND IN EUROPE

2000/2001 figures
Percentage relates to
amount of agricultural
land given over to organic
production. In all cases the
figure is rising - in many
cases, with government
support, at a dramatic rate.

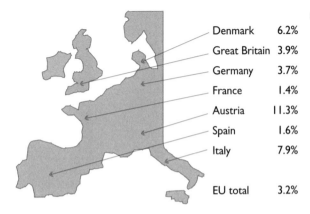

Denmark	6.2%
Great Britain	3.9%
Germany	3.7%
France	1.4%
Austria	11.3%
Spain	1.6%
Italy	7.9%
EU total	3.2%

US STATISTICS

Only 0.3% of all US crop and 0.2% of all US pasture was certified organic in 2001

Hugely successful, they now supply fabric to the burgeoning market for organic clothing. In 2001, buoyed by the project's success, Schleswig-Holstein announced plans to increase the area under organic cultivation.

In Denmark, the government set targets for the organic production of animal feed, dairy and pork products. With government policy behind them, Danish producers invested in building organic capacity and the Danes now have the world's largest per capita consumption of organic food. But it was in exports that Denmark had the real pay-off. When British supermarkets in the late 1990s were desperately seeking organic butter, milk and bacon to supply the exploding demand in the UK for organic food, the Danes were ready and willing to supply. The 'import gap' for organic food is a British national scandal, with 70% of organic supplies imported, compared to less than 45% for conventional food. Once imports are established it can be difficult for UK producers to recapture market share. Indeed, organic dairy farmers were faced with surpluses and low prices when UK production eventually caught up. Danish producers, meanwhile, enjoy strong sales in Scandinavia, Germany, Holland and even the US, supported by an efficient domestic market where 22% of milk sold in Denmark is organic, as well as 33% of all bread.

Italy has 2.5 million organic acres; 25% of all organic land in the EU. Over 400 farms offer "agri-bio" holidays where visitors can relax in organic countryside. Parental concern about BSE and GM food led the government in July 2000 to actively encourage the serving of organic food in school cafeterias, following the example set by the city of Ferrara. In 1994 Ferrara's kindergartens and nursery schools switched to serving organic pasta, bread, rice, beans and tomatoes and soon moved on to organic fruit and vegetables. By 1998 the program was extended to all schools and now 80% of school food is organic. Kids who eat organic as babies and eat organic at school tend to eat organic at home. Shops stock more organic food and prices fall as steady demand brings greater stability to the supply system. A "virtuous circle" is in operation.

In Britain, the "best-value" principle of local authorities has meant price alone has been the criterion for purchasing decisions. Finally, in July 2002 this policy was modified to include environmental and health criteria, offering Britain's schools, hospitals and government canteens the chance to use organic food. The ingredient cost of the average British school dinner is 50¢; the average ingredient cost of a prison meal is $1. But schools that have switched to organic and local food have seen uptake of school meals double from 40% to more than 80%, so the increased ingredient cost is more than offset by reduced labor and other non-food overhead costs.

What took Britain so long? Well, Britain exports more agrichemicals than most. When the interests of parents and consumers clash with those of the British Agrochemicals Association, the Fertilizer Manufacturers Association and the British Pest Control Association it is difficult for civil servants to balance priorities. However, the cost to Britain's farmers, to the environment and to the balance of payments can be seen, with hindsight, to have been enormous – far greater than any savings to the agrichemical industry.

Regenerating Agriculture
Jules Pretty
National Academy Press 1995
ISBN 0-3090524-6-7

PICK 'N' MIX

a little of what you fancy

A military base was noted for its low level of sickness and high level of performance. When asked why, the base commander took the inquirer to the soldiers' mess, where a sergeant was seen standing at the front of the cafeteria line. From time to time he would send a soldier back to replenish his tray of food. "I count the colors," explained the sergeant. "As long as there are four different colors then the soldier eats."

Simplistic as this may be, when set against the complexity of modern nutrition, it has a long and honorable tradition. Cultures from as wide a range of countries as Italy, Lebanon, Scandinavia and Japan accept that it is better to set out a variety of choices than to prescribe a one-size-fits-all diet. In these countries, before the main course, each diner selects from a choice of starters. A healthy appetite will, given the selection, instinctively choose the right balance of foods. Antioxidants, anthyocyanins, phenolic compounds, fish oils, vitamin precursors, digestive aids, liver tonics and other valuable micronutrients are eaten before the diner moves on to the filling carbohydrate and protein part of the meal. In an age before vitamins and supplements, this was how people ensured good nutrition.

Antipasto is the Italian way: before the main dish the table is set with a range of bites

A healthy appetite will instinctively choose the right balance of foods

– anchovies, tuna, olives, artichoke hearts, basil pastes, mushrooms, beans, grilled or raw chicory, celery hearts, fennel, carrots and broccoli. "Bagna Cauda," a warm dipping sauce based on garlic, anchovies and olive oil is the perfect accompaniment to raw vegetable crudités.

In Lebanon, "mezze" does the same thing with a plate of raw vegetables such as radishes, carrots, cucumbers, mint sprigs, peppers, turnip, lettuce and tomatoes, along with parsley-rich tabouli salad, hummus, tahini, falafel, broad beans and pickles.

The "smorgasbord" of Scandinavia sets out a variety of herring dishes, roasted and raw vegetables, grated beetroot or carrot salads, sweet and sour cabbage, all served with wholegrain pumpernickel bread or crispbreads.

Sushi in Japan ensures that the diner gets dietary essentials: digestion-enhancing miso soup, along

Sushi ensures that the diner gets dietary essentials

with seaweed, oily fish, ginger pickle, tofu, daikon radish and umeboshi plums.

With so many different ingredients, "leftover management" is the key to success. By pickling, marinating, grilling and serving cold, salting and other preservation methods, all the dishes can be rolled out every day, ensuring a continuous and varied selection of nutritional foods, without having to prepare them every day from scratch. The healthiest diet mixes and balances all the food groups – carbohydrate, protein and fat.

Even the best ideas can be corrupted. The "smorgasbord" concept can be abused. Yum! Brands, Inc.'s "Fast Food Smorgasbord" in the US aims to rival McDonald's, with multiple franchises – KFC, Taco Bell, Pizza Hut, Long John Silver's and A&W All American Food – all within one restaurant. Say goodbye to those family squabbles in the car over which fast-food outlet to visit. Now everyone can get his or her own favorite fatty, refined junk food under one roof.

- Korean cuisine is considered by nutritionists to be the world's best. This is because it typically consists of about 70% carbohydrate, 17% protein and is very low in fat. By contrast, the typical Western diet is only about 40% carbohydrate and 15% to 20% fat, as well as 15% to 20% sugar.

PACKAGING

a necessary evil?

Banana skins, orange peels and wheat husks are natural packaging; all contain the edible inner part in transit and keep out bugs, dirt and other contaminants.

The earliest forms of "added" packaging used natural materials – banana leaves, corn husks and gourds. All 100% recyclable, they were discarded harmlessly when no longer needed. Willow baskets and terracotta urns were early man-made packaging that enabled the transport of solids and liquids over long distances without loss of quality. They could be reused until they were no longer useable.

Glass, paper and cardboard were the next wave of packaging materials and opened the way for branded, prepacked foods to feed the growing urban population. They were recyclable and, in the case of glass, reuseable. Old newspapers and printers' off-cuts were used to wrap food by grocers – and were used again to light fires, bed animals or insulate pipes. Things have come a long way since then.

In today's cash-rich, time-poor society, packaging has proliferated, creating mountains

Packaging has proliferated, creating mountains of waste in its wake

of waste in its wake. With many ready-to-eat products more energy is used in getting food to our lips than is represented by the food itself.

One sixth of our expenditure on food represents the cost of packaging.

Americans produce 270 million tons of waste a year – 86 million tons are packaging. With collection, landfill and pollution clean-up costs all borne by the taxpayer, this represents a substantial indirect subsidy that masks the real cost of packaging to food processors. It distorts their judgment of how much packaging to use and whether it is recycled, or indeed, even recyclable.

In the United States landfill can continue for some time, but in much of the world there isn't enough landfill space to carry on like this. Something must be done. Fortunately, something is being done. 71% of all cardboard

Taxpayer subsidies mask the real cost of packaging and distorts judgment on types of use

used in the US is recycled, 58% of all newspapers, 57% of steel cans, 57% of yard trimmings, 55% of aluminum cans and one third of all plastic bottles and magazines, with glass containers trailing at only 25%.

The EU aims, as a first step, to double the proportion of packaging that is recycled by 2007, setting a recycling target of between 55% and 70%, up from the current minimum of between 25% and 45%. The new rules will increase targets for recycling glass (60%), paper and board (55%), metals (50%) and plastics (20%).

Already, in Ireland, a plastic carrier bag carries a hefty premium on its cost that helps pay for cleaning up and recycling. This has led rapidly to increased durability and reusability of carrier bags and thus to a much higher rate of reuse. Whole Foods Markets encourages reuse of grocery bags by giving customers 5¢ rebate for every bag reused.

In 1982 Denmark prohibited aluminum cans and encouraged the use of glass containers that could be refilled and reused. Now they are opening the door to aluminum cans again, but with strict recycling conditions.

To produce aluminum, bauxite must be mined. Recycling 1 kg of aluminum saves 8 kg of bauxite, 4 kg of chemical products and 14 kilowatts of electricity. Aluminum can be recycled indefinitely, as reprocessing does not damage its structure. In 2003 the US consumed fifty billion aluminum drinks cans, of which 50% were recycled. This saves energy and raw materials, but is still much lower than Switzerland and Finland at 91%.

Aluminum cans have become thinner and now are made with 40% aluminum.

In Germany, a group of leading organic food processors and wholesalers operate an "Eight for All" scheme where all manufacturers agree to use a standard range of eight different glass jars and bottles. They can then cost-effectively accept returns and reuse each other's packaging.

It is now widely agreed that all participants, from producer to end consumer, must share cradle-to-grave responsibility for the packaging that they produce and use. When producers are liable for material they introduce into the economy, they quickly find ways to minimize the amount they use, and to recycle the rest.

Supermarkets that sell organic food alongside non-organic face the paradox that organic produce requires more packaging as regulations require that it be kept distinct from non-organic produce. One solution is to use biodegradable and compostable trays for organic produce. In Europe, potato starch and cellulose fibers from spruce (paper pulp waste) provide cheap raw materials. Since May 2004, the Earth Fare natural foods supermarket chain in North Carolina pack produce, bakery and delicatessen items in corn-based packaging from Nebraska – it takes 45 days for the packs to break down if sent to one of the 4,000 commercial composting facilities in the USA. Separation remains a problem – when garbage goes to landfill even the compostable material doesn't break down as, once in landfill, materials break down very slowly. Such packaging offers a solution that covers all foods, organic or not

All participants from producer to consumer must share responsibility

– though the buying of food from local suppliers would, of course, massively reduce the huge energy costs of packaging still further.

When hidden subsidies for wasteful practices are eliminated and the true cost of packaging is paid by the users, innovative solutions to reduce, recycle and change the very nature of packaging emerge. All it takes is political will, and one may well wonder why it has all taken so long.

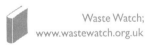

Waste Watch;
www.wastewatch.org.uk

BRAVE NEW WORLD

guess what's coming to dinner

Why has genetic engineering been so controversial? Why is there such concern at the potential risks of eating foods that haven't been properly tested for safety? Most innovation by the food industry is demand-driven, a response to evolving consumer

Most innovation by the food industry is demand-driven

attitudes. Genetic engineering, however, came down from the top. It has been foisted on us. So, have the biotechnology corporations made a hideous mistake?

To answer the question we must look back to the early days of biotechnology, the late 1980s.

With the discovery that it was possible to map genomes and manipulate genetic material, the stock market went wild. Companies came up with all kinds of lucrative plans and were overwhelmed with funds as investors scrambled to be first aboard the gravy train. National governments committed hundreds of millions of dollars of public funds to support research. As with the dot.com boom, nobody could estimate future profits, but nobody wanted to miss out on the huge potential.

Biotechnology promised two main prizes:
A cure for cancer. By the late 1980s investors were losing faith in the ability of drug companies to find a cure for cancer and share prices were falling. Biotechnology's proponents virtually guaranteed a breakthrough. Sadly, the search delivered nothing. British Biotech were UK leaders in the field of cancer research. Valued at $3 billion in 1997, they had dropped in value to $55 million by September 2002, a loss to investors of 98%.

On Wall Street, biotechnology companies can no longer raise funds, no matter how exciting their promises.

Control of the global market for food. Since time immemorial, people have tried to "corner" the market in agricultural commodities. With the promise of genetically modified crops that would yield more, resist diseases, grow in depleted soils, taste better and stay fresh longer, money poured into companies like Monsanto.

The attempt to capture the food and farming markets fared poorly, except in the US and Canada. Monsanto's attempt to dominate the agricultural sector is an example of corporate miscalculation (or deception) on a colossal scale.

Monsanto's patent on their herbicide Roundup was due to expire by 2001. So they inserted a Roundup-resistance gene into soybean and corn plants and came up with "Roundup Ready" crops. Now fields could be sprayed year-round with Roundup without crops being affected. This ensured that farmers would continue to buy Monsanto's brand of generic herbicide. With money raised from gullible investors they bought up the leading seed companies in America, Canada, Argentina and India in order to ensure distribution of their new products. Launched in 1996, sales of GM seed boomed as farmers fell for a marketing pitch that promised higher yields and lower herbicide costs.

What have the results been of the GM experiment in North America?

1. Yields did not increase and often fell – Roundup Ready soybeans yield 6% to 11% less than conventional varieties.

The attempt to capture the food and farming markets with GM food faired poorly outside the US

2. Herbicide use did not decrease and, for many farmers, increased.

3. Gene Pollution – Farmers who didn't buy GM seeds found that cross-pollination had contaminated their crops anyway.

4. Litigation proliferated. Monsanto sent investigators into fields to snip leaf samples from crops. Their lawyers would then sue

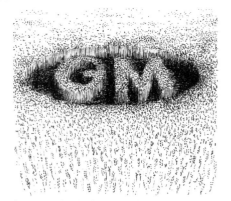

farmers who had traces of Monsanto's DNA growing in their fields. A few farmers hired their own analysts and found that Monsanto's claims were groundless. (This led to a state law in North Dakota requiring that a state analyst must accompany seed company investigators.)

Contamination of non-GM crops undermined their value. Nearly half the US corn supply was affected

Most farmers, when faced with the threat of protracted legal action, meekly paid the more than $10,000 that Monsanto demanded and signed a confidentiality agreement promising not to divulge the terms of the compromise.

5. Rogue herbicide-resistant oilseed rape plants emerged that were immune to three different herbicide groups. Farmers are forced to use more toxic older pesticides such as paraquat to get rid of them.

6. Contamination of non-GM crops undermined their value. The Starlink fiasco, in which an unapproved GM corn variety contaminated nearly half the American corn supply, cost the owners of the seed, Aventis, $1 billion paid out in compensation, with claims continuing as contamination continues.

7. Export markets collapsed and prices fell. It is estimated that GM crops could have cost the US economy $12 billion between 1999 and 2001. There are nearly two million farmers in the US; in 2002 their survival required subsidies of over $150 billion, or $75,000 per farmer.

8. Organic farmers suffered. In Saskatchewan farmers have given up growing organic canola because of contamination. The global market for GM seeds, for which no consumer demand exists, is $4 billion. The global market for organic food, for which real demand exists, is $22 billion.

9. Farmer groups across North America are

united in opposition to the introduction of GM wheat, fearing even worse problems with an important export crop.

10. Under pressure from consumers and farmers, the US Congress is considering legislation to provide for GM labeling, to assign legal liability for the costs of GM disasters to the biotech companies and to protect farmers from legal harassment.

In 2004, Mendocino County in California decided by referendum to ban the growing of GM plants anywhere in the county. Similar initiatives are under way in other states.

With such a negative outcome after only six years of GM crops, the rest of the world is understandably cautious.

In Argentina, Monsanto met farmer resistance – so it abandoned the technology fees and sold farmers GM seeds on long-term credit, with payment after harvest. In 2002, Argentinian farmers could not pay their seed bills and Monsanto had to confiscate farmers' property. It wrote off $2 billion from its balance sheet in the value of the seed companies and $180 million in unpaid debts.

Brazil, which was set to go GM, decided to stay GM-free in order to tap into the lucrative market for non-GM crops in the EU and Japan. In the EU, China, India, Mexico, Sri Lanka, Canada, Thailand, Bosnia, Ecuador, Colombia, Guatemala, Nicaragua, Zambia, Zimbabwe and Mozambique there has been dogged resistance to GM food imports and prolonged wrangling with US trade envoys. Farmers, used to saving seed, are

Many US counties are holding referendums to ban GM farming

reluctant to adopt a technology that prohibits this practice and which has the "Terminator" gene in reserve to enforce dependency on annual seed purchase. The US government is expending scarce diplomatic capital in trying to force GM crops into export markets. Nations facing famine risk reject GM food, given as food aid through the World Food Program.

What future is there for GM crops? Nobody in Europe, Asia, Africa or Latin America wants to eat them. Few farmers want to grow them. Retailers find advantage in guaranteeing their products to be GM free. No investor wants to invest in them. They may still have powerful political support, but the market is unlikely to change its verdict.

• "Perhaps the biggest issue raised by these results is how to explain the rapid adoption of genetically engineered crops when farm financial impacts appear to be mixed or

Retailers find advantage in guaranteeing their products to be GM free

even negative." From *The Adoption of Bio-engineered Crops*, a US Department of Agriculture report, May 2002.

• "If anyone tells you that GM is going to feed the world, tell them that it is not. To feed the world takes political and financial will." Steve Smith, Director of biotech corporation Novartis (now Syngenta), in 2002.

• "When you inject a supply-driven concept into a demand-driven market, it's a recipe for failure." Ron Olson, vice president of General Mills.

Lords of the Harvest
Daniel Charles
Perseus 2003
ISBN 0-7382077-3-X

Seeds of Deception
Jeffrey Smith
Yes! Books 2003
ISBN 0-9729665-8-7

GROW YOUR OWN

when mud doesn't matter

*"Adopt the pace of nature,
her secret is patience."*
Emerson

When I return from my nearby community garden with my home-grown vegetables, I present them to the family and announce proudly: "Look at that, $40 worth of vegetables." To which a legitimate reply would be: "That would only cost $10 at the supermarket!"

So why bother? Even at the minimum wage, the cost in your time, horse manure, tools, seeds and seedlings far exceeds the cost of just buying your vegetables, washed and trimmed, from the supermarket, with no slugs, no flea beetle, no white rot, no blight, no cabbage white butterfly, no backache. But that's if you don't value the rewards of "horticultural therapy."

Growing food for your own table is richly satisfying -- a healthful pursuit for mind, body and spirit. It can be done with the minimum of space in an urban apartment or you can take on a plot at a community garden and get really serious.

A vegetable such as a beet or a cabbage, freshly harvested, lightly cooked or eaten raw, can easily be the central feature of a meal. In a restaurant you'd feel short changed, but at

Growing your own food connects you with the elements

home, a vegetable grower's achievement brings pleasure to all who share it.

Growing your own food connects you with the elements of air, sunshine, earth and water. A tiny seed germinates, sends a tentative few leaves skyward and the gardener nurtures it until harvest. Watching this, learning patience yet being amazed at how rapidly some things can grow, brings a new level of respect for the power of plants. Passing time, the vagaries of weather, the changes of day-length as the seasons go through their cycle, all root us in a deeper reality far from the artificial concerns of the "real" world.

Composting – the creation of soil from waste vegetable materials – is nature's alchemy. Converting base waste materials into pure horticultural gold is the Philosopher's Stone of gardening. The "Rule of Return" is played out

An hour of gardening burns up 50% more calories than gardening, and bone health benefits

in slow motion as discarded vegetable parts, weeds and other "trash" are transformed into crumbly brown compost that promises new fertility and life for the soil. When they move house, many people leave behind fixtures and fittings, but wouldn't dream of abandoning the compost heap. There is a real reward in working with the bacteria and fungi that add so much to the fertility of soil.

Growing your own food is good exercise, too. Like swimming, no part of the body is left unworked by hoeing, raking, digging, pulling weeds and planting seeds. Backache is a concern, but respect for the back's limitations can ensure strengthening and toning without pain. An hour of gardening burns up 345 calories, 50% more than cycling. Bone health benefits both from activity and from exposure to sunlight. A different, deeper rhythm of nature takes over, to which our minds and bodies instinctively respond. It's mind work, too – plants are complex and challenging and learning to understand them is deeply stimulating.

Window boxes and indoor plants are nurseries for learning practical skills, even if you're only growing a tomato plant. But community gardens are even better. Once the soil is in good condition the constant cycle of adding more compost is like a savings account – with a healthy interest rate repaid in tasty fresh vegetables. And there's a social life at community gardens, too: mutual support, friendly advice and the sharing of plants and surpluses.

Pick up a seed catalogue and read it alongside a newspaper. Which one fills you with hope?

• The American Community Gardening Association will advise on locations of existing community gardens and on the establishment and management of new ones. www.communitygarden.org

• You can have the fun of growing vegetables without the responsibility of your own plot of land. WWOOF (World Wide Opportunities on Organic Farms) enables you to help as a volunteer on organic farms around the world. www.wwoof.org

Compost
Clare Foster
Cassell 2002
ISBN 0-3043623-1-X

EDUCATION

grass-root concerns

How important food and nutrition are depends greatly on where you live and what you do.

The average American spends 7% of their income on food and non-alcoholic drink; the average Briton 10% and the average Frenchman 15%. Shopping, cooking and eating occupy one in sixteen of our waking hours. Understanding the importance of food is one of the key "life skills" we should all have acquired as children. Most food education is focused on food safety, avoiding food poisoning from bugs and germs that shouldn't be in food in the first place.

In 12 years of primary and secondary education most children learn nothing about food, nutrition and health apart from tangential references in biology, where the human digestive system and metabolism are studied. Home economics, a study previously restricted to female students, has been widely abandoned as a result of curriculum changes. Many students leave school able to calculate the collision time of two trains travelling at different speeds in opposite directions but unable to boil an egg, or bake a loaf of bread. There has been a marked decline in the number of students who opt to study food science or food technology.

In the four years of medical education that a doctor undergoes before qualification, just four hours are spent studying the subject of nutrition and health. In most hospitals the dietician or nutritionist is a lowly staff member, who is not allowed to diagnose and whose main role is to issue pre-programmed nutritional advice, mostly to diabetics. Hospital food is prepared with little attention to the individual's medical condition.

But children do get information about food. Between the age of two and 12 a Canadian child will see 100,000 television commercials for food. At the age of three one in five American children are making specific brand-name requests for food. Channel One's 12-minute in-classroom broadcast, featuring two minutes of commercials for every 10 minutes of news, is compulsory on 90% of the school days in 80% of the classrooms in 40% of US middle and high schools. Companies pay up to $195,000 for a 30-second ad, knowing that they have a captive audience of eight million students in 12,000 classrooms across the country. Coca-Cola pays schools and supplies educational material in exchange for exclusive rights to place drinks-vending machines in schools. They also lobby to allow students to have carbonated drinks in class.

How can children possibly obtain a balanced view of healthy nutrition in the face of such overwhelming corporate influence?

The Soil Association Demonstration Farms Network helps educate children in the origins of food. The aim is that every child in Britain will have visited an organic farm and been educated in the fundamentals of food production by the age of 12. Children remember 20% of what they are told and 80% of what they do, so farm visits have a real and lasting educational impact. Because organic farms usually have a mixture of crops and livestock the whole picture of food production can be studied. Demonstration farms allow kids to see animals close-up and help them understand the connection between sustainable farming and care of the countryside. They can also buy fresh food from the farm

1 in 5 American children make requests for food brands at age 3

shop, or taste something at the farm café. The challenge is then to encourage an ongoing interest in wholesome fresh food.

In Wisconsin, the Appleton Alternative Central High School gave the school meals contract to a company called Natural Ovens and took out soft drink and snack machines. School meals were nutritionally balanced and included wholegrains and plenty of vegetables. Academic performance improved by one full grade point, violence fell to such an extent that the regular police patrol on duty was withdrawn and put back on the beat. One teacher postponed retirement saying "I love teaching here now – it's why I joined this profession." A delegation from Los Angeles visited the school in 2002 and a year later soft drinks and snack vending machines were withdrawn from all schools in the L.A. area. Similar initiatives have begun in New York and other school districts. Behavioral improvement is almost immediate.

These educated consumers form a bloc that food manufacturers ignore at their peril. In the words of a General Mills executive: "Our research shows that 8% to 9% of American consumers will not buy a product if it contains GM ingredients – that's too large a chunk of our customer base to ignore unless GM offers some real benefits elsewhere." TV food advertising assumes ignorance among consumers. Brand loyalties cost a great deal to develop. Educated consumers will force a change in the values of companies that do not want to lose their expensively acquired customers.

• In June 2002, the UK television company GMTV accepted a £1 million sponsorship deal with McDonald's for its cartoon slot on weekend mornings. Such a deal helps to target junk food at three- to eight-year-old children. A child in that age range eating a McDonald's birthday party meal, choosing a cheeseburger, regular fries (with tomato ketchup), a regular coke and a slice of birthday cake would consume 889 calories, 81g of sugar; 27.7g of fat (11.5g saturated fat) and 1.6g of sodium (equivalent to 4g of salt). For a four- to six-year-old this would be 60% of the maximum total recommended daily intake of saturated fat, 79% more sugar and 128% more salt than the maximum total recommended daily intake. For a seven- to ten-year-old it would be 53% of recommended daily intake of saturated fat, 58% more sugar and 33% more salt.

Stupid White Men ... and Other Sorry Excuses for the State of the Nation
Michael Moore
Regan Books 2002
ISBN 0-0603924-5-2

FROM TOBACCO TO TABASCO

nightshade foods and human health

In the diet of Europe and Asia only one nightshade food was eaten until recent times: the aubergine or eggplant. Other nightshades such as henbane, thorn apple (*datura stramonium*), belladonna and mandrake were well known but their use was restricted to specific medical applications (sedative, anesthetic or poison) or to witchcraft.

Then, in the 1600s and 1700s, food and drug crops based on nightshades were imported from the Americas and, over the past 400 years, have become ubiquitous in the Western diet. These include tobacco, tomatoes, potatoes and chili peppers. It is not surprising that, being nightshades, they were regarded with suspicion at first and were slow to take hold in the European diet. They all contain nicotine in some form, although it goes under different names: solanine (potatoes), tomatine (tomatoes), alpha-solanine (eggplant) or solanadine (chilies and capsicums).

Increasingly, some people are finding that they cannot tolerate nightshades in their diets and that eliminating them helps alleviate a variety of mental, emotional and physical problems. Among them are:

1. People with arthritis — some researchers believe that arthritis is misdiagnosed in

Some people are finding that they cannot tolerate nightshades

people who are in fact just suffering joint aches and swelling arising from consumption of nightshades. One in three arthritics reacts badly to nightshades.

2. Macrobiotics – the macrobiotic diet has always counseled abstinence from nightshades.

3. Children with eczema – for some children, the elimination of nightshades from the diet helps clear eczema, particularly around the mouth.

4. Gastro esophogal reflux disease – consumption of tomatoes can cause a reaction where the stomach contents are pushed back up the esophagus towards the

> One doctor recommends the avoidance of nightshade foods for about half the population

throat with symptoms of heartburn, chest pain, choking while lying down and asthma when sleeping.

5. Quitting smoking – some programs to help people give up cigarettes also recommend giving up nightshades in order to eliminate low-level nicotine intake from food.

6. Blood group diet – Dr. Peter d'Adamo's Blood Type Diet recommends avoidance of nightshade foods for blood types A and B. This represents about half the population.

A Closer Look at Nightshades
Tomatoes

In 1820, Colonel Robert Johnson defied the advice of his physicians ("You will foam and froth at the mouth and double over") and ate tomatoes on the steps of Salem Courthouse, New Jersey, in front of a crowd of 2,000 witnesses. He survived and America slowly began to accept tomatoes as food. Tomatoes really took off as food with the introduction of canning and canned soups – then rose again with the boom in pizza and pasta consumption.

Potatoes

Traditionally, potatoes were kept in paper sacks and sold unwashed. This protected them from direct sunlight. Washing potatoes and selling them in plastic bags allows light to affect the potato and stimulates its production of solanine. In 1976, Britain's Department of Health, concerned about high levels of anencephaly and spina bifida, urged pregnant mothers to wear rubber gloves when preparing potatoes and to discard in their entirety any potatoes that showed signs of greening or of blight (black streaks in the potato). It is not enough to simply remove the discolored part – the entire potato should not be eaten. The solanine in potatoes is four times greater in the skin than in the rest of the potato. The fatal dose of solanine for an adult is 200 mg to 250 mg depending on body weight. Potatoes shouldn't normally contain more than 90 mg of solanine per pound, so it would take more than 2 lbs of potatoes to be fatal. Potatoes that have been properly stored and are from low solanine varieties will only contain 30 mg/lb. In 1996, Britain's Committee on Toxicity stated that potatoes should not be eaten if they still taste bitter after the green parts and sprouts have been removed. However, few people taste-test a raw potato to assess its bitterness.

Peppers

Peppers were rare in the Western diet until the 1980s, when they became widely available in Asian and Tex-Mex cuisine and as hot sauce. Peppers and capsicums contain solanine and solanadine.

Eggplants

Eggplants most resemble in appearance the belladonna nightshade plant that may be their wild ancestor.

What are cholinesterase inhibitors?

The alkaloids in nightshades are cholinesterase inhibitors:

- The chemical that conducts nerve impulses is acetylcholine.
- Acetylcholine is produced by an enzyme: acetyl cholinesterase.
- Nightshade alkaloids interfere with this enzyme.
- The production of acetylcholine declines.
- The nerve endings have to work harder to transmit signals as they don't have the help of sufficient acetylcholine.
- Acetylcholine helps keep the bodily fluids running – reduced levels lead to dryness in the mouth and throat, reduced lubrication of the joints and reduced intestinal secretions, causing constipation.

Before the discovery of chemical pesticides, nicotine was a widely used insecticide. It kills insects by blocking acetylcholine and shutting down their central nervous system. It was replaced by chemical sprays that are cheaper and longer lasting.

Why do people love nightshades?

What is it that makes nightshades so attractive?

Why is it that sometimes only French fries will do, or we are aching for a pizza? Nicotine, in small quantities, by inhibiting the supply of acetylcholine, stimulates increased activity of the acetylcholine receptors in the brain, leading to an increased flow of adrenaline. This in turn increases the heart rate and blood pressure and leads to increased blood glucose levels. A mild increase in energy level is achieved, along with a reduced nervous sensitivity, producing a combination of calmness and stimulation. This provides short-term relief in the face of the stresses and pressures of modern life.

If the nightshade foods were to be introduced to the Western diet today, under current

> If nightshade foods were to be introduced today, it is unlikely they would be permitted

food safety regulations, it is unlikely that they would be permitted to enter the food supply because of their nicotine (solanine) content. Like cigarettes, they slipped into our lifestyle and, despite some voices in opposition, have assumed a major role in our nutrition and health – a role that, in a free society, should be accepted. However, nightshade foods should be understood for what they are and consumed with an awareness of their psychotropic and physical effects.

VITAMINS

preventing prevention

In the US and Europe, for a decade, there has been a determined, unrelenting attempt to stop people from taking preventive medicine in the form of vitamins, supplements and herbal medicines. No issue generates more mail to elected representatives from angry citizens than the attempt to deny them the right to take responsibility for their own health. Yet there has been a steady erosion of this freedom that threatens to hand control to a handful of drug companies.

Remember why this is happening – pharmaceutical companies are in crisis worldwide. The pipeline of new blockbuster drugs is empty. The antibiotic trail has gone cold. Diseases like MRSA show that more powerful drugs create more virulent, resistant bacteria. Profit margins are falling – a Ventolin inhaler sells for $49 in the US, but only $10 in the UK and a knock-off from India sells for $1.50. Medical journals have imposed stringent new ethical rules on publishing research that make the old bogus methods of getting new drugs approved much more difficult – all research undertaken must be published, not just the favorable results. Prescription drugs are responsible for 100,000 deaths in America each year – and that's just the "properly prescribed and administered" ones. GM and biotechnology haven't produced any of the miracle cures

GM and biotech haven't produced any of the miracle cures promised

promised – not one. Medical treatment is now the leading cause of death in the US, with pharmaceutical drugs the main causative factor. The lobbying by drug companies to lower the level at which drugs are prescribed for diastolic blood pressure from 90 to 80 could generate 6,000,000 new medication candidates in the US alone. This is lucrative because every patient on blood pressure drugs then also needs to take daily diuretics, aspirins and anti-ulcer drugs to combat aspirin's side effects. How much simpler if consumers simply ate well and ate less, avoiding the poor arterial tone and plaque build-ups that make high blood pressure a risk for stroke. (It was only a decade or so ago that high diastolic blood pressure was considered to be over 100.)

Long before vitamins were discovered, people knew that certain foods could prevent disease.

Before vitamins were discovered people knew that certain foods could prevent disease

British sailors were known as "limeys" because they regularly ate Vitamin C-rich limes to prevent scurvy. The British Empire depended on a strong navy and healthy sailors. Refining rice removed thiamine (Vitamin B1) and led to widespread beri-beri epidemics in the Orient. Refining corn led to pellagra outbreaks due to niacin (Vitamin B3) deficiency. Vegetarians in particular should avoid refined grains and bread as meat is the fallback source of these and many other vitamins and minerals. It could be argued that the increase in meat consumption parallels the refinement of cereal foods and reflects the instinctive desire to obtain missing vitamins and minerals from some other food source.

Most of the research and classification of vitamins and minerals took place in the 1930s. Since then a deeper understanding of human metabolic processes and the role of other trace elements has led to discoveries of phytochemicals, other elements in food that play an important role in health. Lutein (from kiwi fruit, green vegetables and marigold petals) contributes to good eyesight. Anthocyanins (from red and purple foods such as blueberries, red cabbage and grapes) have antioxidant properties and help prevent cancer. Rutin (found in buckwheat and apples) helps blood pressure and relieves hemorrhoids. The "father of medicine" Hippocrates wrote, "Let your food be your medicine," and listed the medicinal properties of over 400 different foods and herbs.

Levels of vitamins, minerals and phytochemicals in food fall when it is grown with agrichemicals. Organic food consistently shows significantly higher levels.

There should never be a need for vitamins or supplementation if one consumes a balanced diet of organic foods and leads a stress-free lifestyle with good levels of activity. But for the 99.9% of the population who can't lay claim to the above ideal situation, there are bound to be occasional deficiencies that vitamin, mineral and herb supplementation can rectify.

Disease is the ultimate result of a deficiency in vitamins and minerals. But absence of disease is not health – for positive health and vitality supplementation can make the difference between feeling average and feeling truly alive.

With the right dietary choices, an understanding of the symptoms of nutritional deficiencies and access to healthy organic food, it is possible to prevent disease. Vitamins, minerals and concentrated phytochemicals extracted from plant sources enable us to prevent the consequences of dietary failings.

So why are drug companies keeping up the pressure to criminalize the self-administration of vitamins?

They don't want to suppress the vitamin and mineral business. They want to take it over. They've seen sales of complementary and alternative medicine heading steadily upwards while drug sales are in freefall. They can make the raw materials that many vitamin and supplement formulators use but that's the commodity end of the scale – now they want to get in at the retail end. The drug that the pharmaceutical industry is hopelessly hooked on is regulation – they are most viable when lobbying a few bureaucrats determines which drugs (or herbs and vitamins) get used, what price they sell at and where they can be on sale. Once supplements are regulated and only big companies can afford to secure product approvals, they can write their own ticket.

The right to practice preventive medicine is not just a health issue; it's a question of the fundamental freedom of human beings to take responsibility for their own health.

SOME CONCLUSIONS

Dateline New York 2012 – The United Nations World Food and Health Organization (WFHO) has published its State of the World Report.

Key data: The world's population has reached a plateau at 10 billion. Life expectancy in all the world's nations continues to rise, with a global average of 80 years. Levels of heart disease, cancer, obesity and diabetes are in steep decline, ensuring a greatly improved quality of life for the aged. Infant and childhood mortality has plummeted. The ongoing program of converting hospitals into luxury apartments continues, with 7,000 hospitals converted to other uses in the year 2011. The number of the world's citizens employed in agriculture continues to increase, as does the proportion of part-time agriculturalists. Farm sizes continue to reduce, with 40 acres the optimal economic unit. Grain reserves now stand at 400 days. Starvation has gone the way of smallpox – totally eradicated. Land retirement continues as meat consumption worldwide falls to an annual average 13 pounds per person. GNP per person has risen with the reduction of military capacity, transferring death-creating investment across to money-saving, planet-saving technologies. Emigration from Europe and North America continues to infuse Africa, Asia and Latin America with the capital and skills from returning immigrants. The world's economy continues to thrive since the Global Trade Justice Agreement of 2006 that led to the abolition of all US, EU and Japanese agricultural subsidies and protectionism following the Cairns Group Ultimatum of 2005. McDonald's recently announced that its sales of organic vegetarian burgers now outstrip beefburger sales by six to one, with wholewheat buns representing more than half of all buns sold. Monsanto, whose genomics seed division has continued to come up with naturally bred, landrace seed varieties tailored to the precise soil and climate requirements of the world's regions, announced record profits and commended the Small Farmers Seed Saving Program for ensuring ideal genetic traits are maintained.

Fantasy? Not a bit of it. Nothing in this optimistic scenario should stretch the credulity of anyone who's read this little book. We have the technologies to avoid the immutable forces that lead us to starvation, obesity, disease and environmental degradation.

But here's the problem. We suffer a distorted food and agriculture system where powerful forces coerce and cajole governments to work against the public interests. Nobody really gains much from it. We didn't ask for the system we got – it has been sold as delivering the greatest goods, but in practice it demands ever-increasing subsidy and brings obesity, new more virulent bacterial diseases, increasing dependence on chemical fungicides, insecticides and herbicides as well as a cocktail of antibiotics, genetically engineered hormones, drugs and adulterants in our food and environment.

We need a new kind of accounting that counts all the costs, both in terms of shareholder profit and the rise in ill health. Nowhere on the national account are the heartache of the bereaved, loss of earning power, amputation, blindness and agonizing pain considered. If they were, we'd be in a very different situation with food.

Is cheap food worth the ill health that is its concomitant? The environmental destruction? The excessive use of fossil fuels? The risk of global warming and increasingly violent weather and flooding? Do we really want our children to enter puberty in hormonal turmoil, brought on by consumption of endocrine-disrupting chemicals in unpredictable interactions with the hormone imbalances inherent in obesity? The inevitable result in the longer run will be evolutionary degeneration. Surely this wasn't part of the deal?

But it's happened. Inexorable, focused pressure on governments around the world means the richest 20% of the world's population suffer chronic obesity disease and the poorest 20% starve. The middle 60% aren't doing that well, either – except, that is, for a rapidly growing minority who engage in "joined-up thinking" about food, diet and farming. If you do the arithmetic properly, i.e. from the perspective of society, eating unsubsidized, locally and organically grown wholesome food free of artificial additives is the answer for our own bodies – and ultimately, for our planet.

REFERENCES

References: general

The Great Food Gamble by John Humphrys
Chivers Press Ltd. 2002 ISBN: 075401692
Food Nations by Warren Belasco, Philip Scranton
Routledge 2001 ISBN: 0415930774
The Botany of Desire: A Plant's-Eye View of the World
by Michael Pollan
Random House Trade 2002 ISBN: 0375760393
*The World is Not For Sale: Farmers Against Junk
Food* by Jose Bove, Francois Dufour, Gilles Luneau
(Translator), Anna de Casparis
Verso 2001 ISBN: 1859846149
*Slow Food: Collected Thoughts on Taste, Tradition,
and the Honest Pleasures of Food*
by Carlo Petrini, Benjamin Watson, Slow Food
Movement
Chelsea Green Publishing Company 2001 ISBN:
1931498016
Food Politics by Marion Nestle
University of California Press 2003 ISBN: 052020677
Silent Spring by Rachel Carson
Mariner Books 2002 ISBN: 0618249060
State of the World 2004 by Worldwatch Institute
W.W. Norton & Company ISBN: 0-393-32539-3
www.worldwatch.org/pubs/sow/2004/
Living Planet Report 2002 by The World Wildlife Fund
www.panda.org

Useful websites

British Farm Standards: www.littleredtractor.org.uk
Center For Food Safety: www.centerforfoodsafety.org
Corporate Watch: www.corporatewatch.org.uk
Corp Watch: www.corpwatch.org
Department of the Environment, Food and Rural
Affairs: www.defra.gov.uk
Earth Council: www.ecouncil.ac.cr
Food and Agriculture Organization of the United
Nations: www.fao.org
Footprint: www.iclei.org
Forum for the Future: www.forumforthefuture.org.uk
Friends of the Earth: www.foe.org
Local Harvest: www.localharvest.org

National Center for Appropriate Technology:
www.ncat.org

National Family Farm Organization: http://www.nffc.net

Organic Consumers Association:
www.organicconsumers.org

Organic Trade Association: http://www.ota.com/
index.html

Organic Center for Education and Promotion: http:
//www.organic-center.org

People for the Ethical Treatment of Animals:
www.goveg.com

Rachel's Environment and Health Weekly:
www.rachel.org

Soil Association: www.soilassociation.org

Sustain: www.sustainweb.org

Sustainable Development Gateway: www.sdgateway.net

Sustainable Energy and Economy Network:
www.seen.org

United State Department of Agriculture:
www.fas.usda.gov

Vegetarian Resource Group: www.vrg.org

Waste Watch: www.wastewatch.org.uk

World Health Organization: www.who.int.en

Worldwatch Institute: www.worldwatch.org

World Wildlife Fund: www.panda.org

Znet Biotech Watch: http://www.zmag.org/
biotechwatch.htm

References: Chapters

Pop Tarts, Ding Dongs, Twinkies and Civilization •
"Obesity is changing human shape." BBC Online, Sept.
9, 2002. News report from the British Association's
science festival, Leicester.

Why Organics • The Worthington Study report.
Source: "Nutritional Quality of Organic Versus
Conventional Fruits, Vegetables and Grains" by Virginia
Worthington, M.S., Sc.D., C.N.S. published in *The
Journal of Alternative and Complementary Medicine*,
Vol. 7, No. 2, 2001 (pp. 161-173) • Research by
Prof. Jules Pretty:."Food Security through Sustainable
Agriculture." Paper for Novartis Foundation for
Sustainable Development Symposium "Nutrition and
Development." Basel, Switzerland Nov. 30, 2000:
www.novartisfoundation.com/en/symposia/2000/
index.htm (downloadable PDF) • Compassion in
World Farming: http://www.ciwf.org.uk. "CIWF seeks
to achieve the global abolition of factory farming and
the adoption of agricultural systems which meet the
welfare needs of farm animals in the belief that this
will also benefit humanity and the environment." • Soil
degradation: "Global Environment Outlook 3 – Past,
Present and Future Perspectives." United Nations
Environment Program 2002: http://geo.unep-wcmc.org.

Obesity • Obesity figures: 1999 estimate by the US
Centers for Disease Control and Prevention, the

body established to oversee America's health policy. www.cdc.gov/nccdphp/dnpa/obesity/defining.htm.

Very Fast Food • UK food poisoning figures from Food Standards Agency *Attitudes to Food Report 2001* • Obesity figures from WHO report Oct. 30, 2002.

Intensive Agriculture • Soil erosion: GEO3, UNEP, 2002. More details at: http://geo.unep-wcmc.org.

The (Not-so?) Green Revolution • Rise in number of hungry people: www.southcentre.org/publications/occasional/paper04/paper4-04.htm. This refers to Rosset, Collins and Lappe 2000 "Lessons from the Green Revolution: Do We Need New Technology To End Hunger?" in *Tikkun Magazine* Vol 15, No 2 pp 52-56, March/April 2000. • Number of children dying from malnutrition refers to the UNICEF figure at: www.unicefusa.org/malnutrition/ • Useful figures at: www.worldhunger.org/articles/global/ray.htm#Table%201.

Tastes Familiar • In August 1995 The Federation of American Societies for Experimental Biology (FASEB) presented to FDA the final report on its FDA-commissioned review of the safety of the food ingredients monosodium glutamate (MSG) and other free glutamates. On the basis of this report the FDA extended the requirement to label monosodium glutamate to requiring foods containing it, such as "autolyzed yeast" or "soy sauce" to add the phrase "contains glutamate," so that consumers could have some idea of how much glutamate they are consuming. http://vm.cfsan.fda.gov/~lrd/msg.html.

Sweet Nothings • Aspartame reported side effects include headaches, nausea, abdominal cramps, vision changes, diarrhea and seizures. Full listings at: www.mac-archive.com/ns/side.html and www.321recipes.com/symptoms.html.

The American Footprint • www.nrcs.usda.gov has more information on the Natural Resources Inventory.

The Farmer Feeds Them All • The Economic Research Service of the USDA reports that in 2001, about 0.3% of all US cropland and 0.2% of all US pasture was certified organic. www.ers.usda.gov/Data/organic • National Family Farm Organization: http://www.nffc.net.

Pesticides • The Pesticides Residues Committee was established to advise the Food Standards Agency and the Pesticides Safety Directorate on pesticides in food. They test 35-45 different foodstuffs each year, taking 4,000 samples, doing 90,000 individual tests at a government-funded cost of £2 million. In Nov. 2002 they recommended that fruit and vegetables – particularly potatoes – should be peeled before giving them to young children. • Organic farming permits the use of "Bordeaux mixture" a copper sulphate compound used as a fungicide and "rotenone" an extract of derris roots used for insect control. Before using these "last resort" chemicals an organic farmer must justify such as to their certifying body and show what steps have been taken to prevent a recurrence of the problem that led to the need for chemical intervention.

Energy • Ethanol study: Professor David Pimentel, of the Cornell University College of Agriculture and Life Sciences. He chaired a US Dept of Energy panel that investigated the energetics, economics and environmental aspects of ethanol production. His article, "Limits of Biomass Utilization," is in the *Encyclopedia of Physical Science and Technology*: 18 Volume Set Robert A. Meyers (Ed) Academic Press, ISBN: 0122269306.

Organophosphates • "Mad cow disease" theory: Mark Purdey is a Somerset farmer who refused to use organophosphate warble fly treatments on his cattle. They did not develop BSE. His most recent article in Science of Total Environment Oct. 7, 2002; 297(1-3): 1-19 "Transmissible spongiform encephalopathies: a family of etiologically complex diseases – a review." M. Bounias, M. Purdey. Mark Purdey's website: www. purdeyenvironment.com • The 1997 Health and Safety Executive study was aimed specifically at assessing head lice treatments. • Monsanto's Roundup herbicide is an organophosphate, which would normally mean that it is an inhibitor to the enzyme cholinesterase and causes nerve system damage. However Monsanto claim that it is "safe as table salt." Action by the New York State Attorney General in 1997 required Monsanto to cease from describing Roundup as "safe" or "environmentally friendly."

Estrogen • Doctor Vyvyan Howard - Senior Lecturer In Fetal And Infant Toxicopathology at Liverpool University. *Endocrine Disrupters: Environmental Health and Policies* (Environmental Science and Technology Library) Luc Hens (Editor), Vyvyan C. Howard (Editor), Polyxeni Nicolopoulou-Stamati (Editor). Kluwer Academic Publishers; ISBN: 0792370562 • Another interesting title to read is *Our Stolen Future*, Theo Colborn, Abacus 1997 ISBN 0333901649.

Genetically Modified Foods • Monsanto, spun off by Pharmacia in Aug. 2001, is one of the leading companies in genetic engineering and agriculture. Their main product is commodity crop seeds that have been engineered to be resistant to their Roundup herbicide. • Aventis, a Swiss pharmaceutical giant, has an agrochemical division, which produced Starlink, which contaminated US corn supplies and led to the most expensive food recall ever. Their products are resistant to Liberty, their proprietary herbicide brand.

Animal Welfare • 2012 animal rearing directives: The Council of Ministers agreed Directive 99/74/EC that will ban battery cages in 2012 but introduces phased implementation, beginning with an increase in the space allowance for caged birds taking effect from Jan. 1, 2003. More details: www.defra.gov.uk/corporate/publications/ pubcat/cvo/1999/chapter5.pdf • People for Ethical Treatment of Animals (PETA) campaigns against the abuse of animals in food production, entertainment and fashion. They seek the enforcement of animal welfare legislation, which exists in the US and the UK but is implemented halfheartedly: www.peta.org.

Functional Foods • Nutritional needs: a survey by HealthFocus, an Atlanta, Georgia market research firm, showed that 3 out of 4 thought that their own nutritional needs are different from anyone else's. This makes the "one size fits all" approach of functional food difficult to market on a wide scale. Functional food market report: www.healthfocus.net/function.htm.

Antibiotics • Irradiation with Cobalt-60, also known as "cold pasteurization," involves placing highly radioactive Cobalt-60 (also used in cancer treatments) in a "gun" directed at food. The gamma rays kill all bacteria in the food after a period of time. "Radiolytic by-products," novel substances about which nothing is known, are created during irradiation and are the main cause for concern about the use of this technology as a way of dealing with pathogens in food.

Additives • The 1984 Food Labeling Regulations introduced E numbers into British food labeling. The 25% "compound ingredient rule" is part of the same legislation. • E numbers come in categories, which are E100-180 = Colors; E200-252 = Preservatives; E260-297 = Acidities; E300-385 = Antioxidant; E400-429 = Thickeners; E430-499 = Emulsifiers; E620-640 = Flavor Enhancer; E950-967 = Sweeteners.

Wholegrains • Kuala Lumpur Lunatic Asylum: "Rice and beriberi: Preliminary report of an experiment conducted at the Kuala Lumpur Lunatic Asylum" by W. Fletcher. Lancet Journal 1907; i:1776-1779. It was found that patients who consumed brown rice experienced relief from the symptoms of beriberi, confirming that it was a nutritional deficiency disease. In medical research circles this was credited with being the first recorded randomized controlled trial in human subjects.

Nutrition and Food Quality • For 60 years, McCance and Widdowson's *The Composition of Foods* has been the authoritative source of information about the nutritional value of foods consumed in the UK. McCance and Widdowson's *The Composition of Foods*, Sixth summary edition. Cambridge: Royal Society of Chemistry, ISBN: 0-85404-428-0. Purchase from the Royal Society of Chemistry: http://www.rsc.org/is/books/comp_food.htm • Document No. 264: was a Senate Report on Farmland Mineral Depletion. It looked at the consequences of the Dust Bowl and the decline in fertility of prairie soils. It also looked at the implications of this decline in fertility on food quality, particularly the mineral content of the American diet. • Iron deficiency report 2000: The connection made was that iron in blood, as hemoglobin, carries oxygen to the brain and the rest of the body. Without oxygen, the brain functions less efficiently as it cannot metabolize glucose (50% of the body's glucose consumption occurs in the brain). Other symptoms include general weakness, fatigue, brittle nails, paleness and loss of appetite.

Brain Food • Fish oil and dyslexia: Jacqueline B. Stordy. "Dark adaptation, motor skills, docosahexaenoic acid, and dyslexia." *American Journal of Clinical Nutrition*, Vol. 71 (suppl), January 2000, pp. 323S-26S • Details on fish oils and dyslexia are on the Dyslexia online magazine: http://www.dyslexia-parent.com/mag38.html • "Free radicals:" these are atoms or groups of atoms that have odd (unpaired) numbers of electrons. The free electrons cause them to react with other molecules in the body and if they react with DNA or cell membranes they can cause cell damage and cell death. Antioxidants such as beta-carotene and vitamins C and E interact with free radicals and neutralize them, preventing them from causing reactive damage to healthy cells.

Hydrogenation of Fat • In 1994, the Committee on Medical Aspects of Food and Nutrition Policy (COMA) published a report on Nutritional Aspects of Cardiovascular Disease. It recommended that no more than 35% of food energy intake should come from fat. Suggested proportions of fat in the diet: Monounsaturated fatty acids: 40%; Polyunsaturated fatty acids: 20%; Trans fatty acids: 6%; Saturated fatty acids: 34% • The Willett Report: In 1980 Prof Walter Willett at the Harvard School of Public Health launched a study of 67,000 nurses who kept detailed dietary records over 12 years. He chose nurses because they are trained in accurate record-keeping. He then analyzed their dietary patterns in the context of their health status. Much valuable nutritional information has come out of this ongoing study, in addition to establishing a significant link between hydrogenated fat consumption and a number of degenerative conditions. • Report: Willett, W. C. et al., "Consumption of Trans-Fatty Acids in Relation to Risk of Coronary Heart Disease Among Women." Society for Epidemiology Research, Annual Meeting, June 1992, Abstract 249 53. Willett, W. C. et al., "Intake of Trans Fatty Acids and Risk of Coronary Heart Disease Among Women." Lancet Journal 341:581-585, 1993 54. www.heall.com/body/healthupdates/food/hydrogenatedfat.html • An update report on hydrogenated fat and trans-fats available from: www.hsph.harvard.edu/reviews/transfats.html • Sustain July 2001 report: "From TV Dinners — What's being served up by the advertisers?" ISBN: 1-90306016-8. Order from www.sustainweb.org.

Microwaves • Baby formula report: Lita Lee Ph.D reported in the Dec. 9, 1989, *Lancet Journal*. Microwaves and hemoglobin levels: report conducted by Swiss biologist Dr. H.U. Hertel in collaboration with Professor Bernard Blanc at the Swiss Federal Institute of Biochemistry of the University of Lausanne. They sought funding from the Swiss Government, which was refused on the grounds that the experiment would be a waste of time and unnecessary use of lab animals. They then performed a scaled-down study that identified the changes in blood quality. Blanc, B. H./Hertel, H. U. (1992): "Comparative study about the influence on man by food prepared conventionally and in the microwave-oven." Raum & Zeit Special Nr.6, Ehlers, Sauerlach. For more details see www.curezone.com/art under the title: "Are Microwave Ovens A Source Of Danger?" • Russian microwave ban: research leading to the ban carried out at the Institute of Radio Technology at Klinsk, Byelorussia. Among effects of microwaving that led to a ban were: creation of d-Nitrodiethanolamine (a cancer-causing agent), creation of cancer-causing agents within dairy products and cereals, formation of free radicals in root vegetables, digestive and blood disorders in consumers of microwaved food, reduced nutritional content, destruction of nucleoproteins in meats. The 1976 ban was lifted by Gorbachev as part of Perestroika process.

Vegetarians • Realeat, founded by Gregory Sams, were the manufacturers of the first VegeBurger™. The Realeat Survey is demographically representative, conducted at 200 sampling points across the UK. It has shown that vegetarianism has doubled from 2.1% of the population in 1984 to 5% in 1999. 45% of respondents said they were eating less meat. Details at: www.chaos-works.com/index2.html?/vegeburger6.html. • Isaac Bashevis Singer: 1978 Nobel Laureate in Literature, Polish American author.

Fasting • More information at: www.healthy.net and www.freedomyou.com.

Foreign Climes • European organic land: provisional statistics, Sept 2002 from www.organic-europe.net. Pick 'n' Mix • Korean cuisine: *The Cambridge World History of Food* by Kenneth Kiple, Kriemhild Conee Omelas (Ed.) 2000 ISBN 0521402166

Packaging • Danish aluminum ban: The Danish government bowed to EU complaints in January 2002, announcing that the 20-year-old ban would end on condition that retailers charged a deposit of 1.50 Danish crowns (23 US cents) to ensure customers returned empty cans.

Brave New World • "Seeds of Doubt – North American Farmers' Experiences of GM Crops." Soil

Association report Sept 2002 ISBN 0-905200-89-6.
Summary and downloadable version available from:
www.soilassociation.org.
Education • A schedule of 1999 percentage expenditure
on food and non-alcoholic drinks in selected
countries worldwide is at: www.ers.usda.gov/briefing/
CPIFoodAndExpenditures/Data/table97.htm •
• Figures relating to McDonald's birthday meal: The
Food Commission, June 2002 • Dietary reference
values, from which the Recommended Daily Allowance
(RDA) for various food groups and substances are set,
are established by the government's Committee on
Medical Aspects of Food Policy (COMA).

ABOUT THE AUTHOR

Craig Sams is one of the senior figures in the
organic community in the United Kingdom.
Born in the US, he now lives in the UK, where
he is the Chairman of the Soil Association
and the policymaking heart of the organic
movement in the UK, as well as its main
certification body. Craig is the creator of
the Whole Earth organic grocery brand, and,
more recently, of the Green & Black's brand
of organic chocolate. Setting up an organic
cocoa project in Belize is Craig's proudest
achievement, as it has had a transformative
effect on the economy of the southern part of
the country.

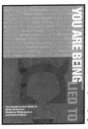

YOU ARE BEING LIED TO
The Disinformation Guide to Media Distortion, Historical Whitewashes and Cultural Myths
Edited by Russ Kick
This book proves that we are being lied to by those who should tell us the truth: the government, the media, corporations, organized religion and others who want to keep the truth from us.
Oversized Softcover • Cultural Studies / Political Science & Government • 400 Pages
$24.95   ISBN 0-96641007-6

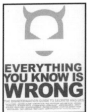

EVERYTHING YOU KNOW IS WRONG
The Disinformation Guide to Secrets and Lies
Edited by Russ Kick
Do you get the feeling that everything you know is wrong? You'll find hard, documented evidence including revelations never before published on the most powerful institutions and controversial topics in the world.
Oversized Softcover • Cultural Studies / Political Science & Government • 352 Pages
$24.95   ISBN 0-9713942-0-2

ABUSE YOUR ILLUSIONS
The Disinformation Guide to Media Mirages and Establishment Lies
Edited by Russ Kick
A stunning line-up of investigative reporters, media critics, independent researchers, academics, ex-government agents and others who blow away the smoke and smash the mirrors that keep us confused and misinformed.
Oversized Softcover • Cultural Studies / Political Science & Government • 360 Pages
$24.95   ISBN 0-9713942-4-5

50 THINGS YOU'RE NOT SUPPOSED TO KNOW
By Russ Kick
Russ Kick has proved himself a master at uncovering facts that "they" would prefer you never hear about: government cover-ups, scientific scams, corporate crimes, medical malfeasance, media manipulation and other knock-your-socks-off secrets and lies.
Trade Paperback • Social Science / Popular Culture • 128 Pages
$9.95   ISBN 0-9713942-8-8

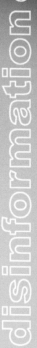
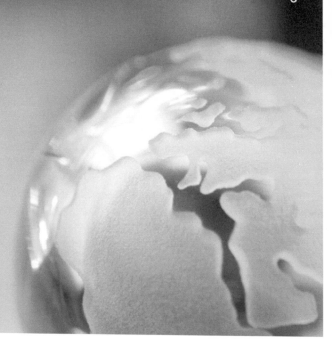

The Little Earth Book

James Bruges

disinformation

The Little Earth Book
James Bruges • Paperback • Environmental Studies /
Political Science & Government
192 Pages • $9.95 • ISBN 0-9729529-2-6

The Earth is now desperately vulnerable, and so are we. This gift-priced-and-sized book contains original, stimulating mini-essays about what is going wrong with our planet – and how to save it. It is pithy, yet well-referenced, wry, deadly serious and in an all-new U.S. edition—the U.K. edition has sold over 40,000 copies! Researched and written by eminent British architect **James Bruges**, The Little Earth Book is an inspiring call to action, a mind-boggling collection of mini-essays on today's most important environmental concerns, from global warming and poisoned food to economic growth, Third World debt, microbes and nanotechnology.

The style is light, undogmatic and sure-footed, explaining complex issues with easy language, illustrations and cartoons. Ideas are developed chapter by chapter, yet each one stands alone. It is an easy browse — equally at home at the bedside table, in the bathroom or in a briefcase.

The Little Earth Book provides hope, with new ideas and examples of people swimming against the current, of bold ideas that work in practice. Packed with easy-to-digest information, James Bruges spells out, clearly, concisely and with alarming documentation just what we're up against and what must be done.

Environmental disasters have left 80 million people as refugees
Already a third of the planet's natural wealth has been lost
90% of the Earth's fresh water supply is consumed by industry

A third of the world is at war
30 million people in Africa are HIV positive
More than 150 countries use torture
Cars kill 2 people every minute …

50 FACTS THAT SHOULD CHANGE THE WORLD

Jessica Williams

50 Facts
That
Should
Change
The World

SEPTEMBER 2004

By Jessica Williams

Trade Paperback

Current Affairs / Popular Culture

352 Pages

$14.95

ISBN 0-9729529-6-9

A third of the world's obese people live in the developing world.

More people can identify the golden arches of McDonald's than the Christian cross.

There are 27 million slaves in the world today.

50 Facts That Should Change The World is a series of snapshots of life in the 21st century. From the inequalities and absurdities of the so-called developed world to the vast scale of suffering wreaked by war, famine and AIDS in developing countries, it paints a picture of incredible contrasts. These are the facts YOU need to know.

This book contains an eclectic selection of facts that address a broad range of global issues. Each is followed by a short essay explaining the story behind the fact, fleshing out the bigger problem lurking behind the numbers. Real-life stories, anecdotes and case studies help to humanize the figures and make clear the human impact of the bald statistics.

The facts paint a picture of a world of inequality: unheard-of and often ludicrous prosperity living alongside crippling poverty. Some of the facts will make you rethink things you thought you knew. Some illustrate long-term, gradual changes in our society. Others concern local issues that people face in their everyday lives. Many will shock.

All of the facts remind us that whether we like to think of it or not, the world is interconnected and civilization is a fragile concept. *50 Facts That Should Change The World* will confront us with some of the hard facts about our civilization, and what we can do about them.

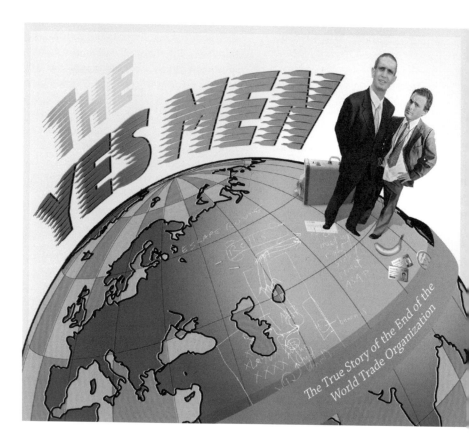

THE YES MEN

The True Story of the End of the
World Trade Organization

This is the companion book to *The Yes Men*, a United Artists movie coming late summer 2004. It follows two anti-corporate activist-pranksters as they impersonate the World Trade Organization on TV and at business conferences around the world.

The story begins with Andy and Mike setting up a website that looks just like that of the World Trade Organization. Some visitors don't notice the site is a fake, and send e-mail invitations meant for the real WTO. Mike and Andy play along with the ruse and soon find themselves attending important functions as WTO representatives.

Delighted to speak as the organization they oppose, Andy and Mike don thrift-store suits and set out to shock their unwitting audiences with darkly comic satires on global free trade. Weirdly, the experts don't notice the joke and seem to agree with every terrible idea the two can come up with.

Exhausted by their failed attempts to shock, Mike and Andy change their strategy completely, and take a whole new approach for one final lecture.

The book is lavishly illustrated in full color throughout, featuring photographs of Mike and Andy getting ever deeper into their assumed identities. Also liberally dispensed are many of the hilarious email exchanges between the Yes Men and various officials and individuals around the world who have asked their advice on issues of world trade.

The Yes Men

By The Yes Men • Trade Paperback • SEPTEMBER 2004
Current Affairs / Political Science & Government
192 Pages • $14.95 • ISBN 0-9729529-9-3

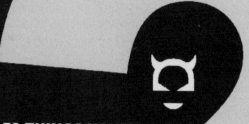

50 THINGS YOU'RE NOT SUPPOSED TO KNOW

RUSS KICK

50 THINGS YOU'RE NOT SUPPOSED TO KNOW – VOLUME 2

By Russ Kick • Trade Paperback • NOVEMBER 2004
Popular Culture / Current Affairs
128 Pages • $9.95 • ISBN 1-932857-02-8

Just in time for 2004's Christmas parties and other holiday get-togethers, **Russ Kick** delivers a second round of stunning information, forgotten facts and hidden history. The first volume was the gift to give and get for the holiday season of 2003; surprising, shocking and controversial, the "things" in *Volume 2* will make 2004's holiday parties sizzle with debate over Kick's revelations — all thoroughly researched and documented.

Sized for quick reference, filled with facts, illustrations and graphic evidence of lies and misrepresentations, *Fifty Things You're Not Supposed To Know— Volume 2* presents the vital, often omitted details on human health hazards, government lies, secret history and warfare excised from your school-books and nightly news reports.

Russ Kick and The Disinformation Company have published five successful books together since 2001. Each one has become a bestseller, establishing Russ as the leader in gathering and disseminating the hidden history, forgotten facts, secret stories and covert cover-ups that "they" don't want you to know!

Ever feel like you're being kept in the dark? Do you feel like the facts and history you rely on might not be the truth, the whole truth and nothing but?

NOTES